Praise for *Healing 1*

"Listen to Avital's authentic, inspiring voice! Springing from the soul, she shares her story of not accepting an "incurable disease" sentence. The stories of all those in this book are powerful reminders to not readily accept limitations that others put on us due to health issues."

—Anita Sanchez, PhD
CEO, Sanchez Tennis & Associates
and best-selling author of *The Four Sacred Gifts*

"Fascinating to read, life-changing to contemplate. These firsthand accounts of the impossible becoming not only possible but the new norm are helping in countless ways to move the whole planet to a greater state of awareness. Anyone facing life lessons about health and well-being would do well to read this book and take its message to heart. We are far more powerful than we know."

—Asha Nayaswami
Author and lecturer

"Avital's own journey of healing, as well as the true stories of healing recounted in this book, creates an easily digestible and powerful resource inspiring us to break through any health issue we're dealing with, no matter how big or small. This book is a catalyst of transformation to help you understand that your breakthroughs in healing can be created by you as you tap into your infinite power and live these spiritually evolved principles. The time is now. Create!"

—Chris Burns
Founder of Becoming Your Greatest Possible Self

"With love, wisdom, and compassion, Avital reminds us that we all have the power to help our minds, bodies, and souls heal themselves—and that no matter what we are going through or experiencing, we can give ourselves this gift. She brilliantly shows how when we are in sync with ourselves we can indeed be blessed, happy, and healthy. Bravo!"

—Gerry Foster
President, GerryFosterBranding.com
and creator of the Big Brand Formula

"If you want to be successful in life, read this book and get inspired to make it happen!"

—Jill Lublin
Four-time best-selling author, international speaker,
and master publicity strategist

"This book is filled with deeply inspiring stories of people who take charge of their health by taking charge of their minds and their bodies. Every one of us deserves to thrive, and Avital gives us a beautiful set of road maps to attain vibrant good health."

—Kit Tennis, PhD
Director of Conscious Organizational Evolution
at Sanchez Tennis & Associates

"Excellent. Balanced. Thought provoking. Inspiring. Avital Miller writes her interviews in ways that stimulate the reader to trust their own intuition, remembering that we are each unique. We each carry dis-ease and heal in our own unique ways. This book is a tapestry of healing stories and methods."

—Janet Lane, MS Clinical Psychology
Director of Children's Ministries at Hope Lutheran Church

"I felt a connection to many of the stories shared within the conversations in this book. Taking preventative actions to secure better health by taking responsibility of our thoughts, actions and environment are keys to realize that Healing Happens."

—Michelle Mras
Inspirational keynote speaker and author

"Healing Happens returns the responsibility for our well-being back to where it belongs—to our own life force, willpower, positive choices, and our desire to grow. Thank you, Avital, for reminding us through this masterful book of our immense potential to heal ourselves."

—Lila Devi
Author and founder of Spirit-in-Nature Essences

"A straight-from-the-heart book that goes straight to the heart."

—Harbeen Arora, PhD
Global chairperson, ALL Ladies League and Women Economic Forum,
founder of BIOAYURVEDA, and author of *Creative Living*

Healing Happens

STORIES OF HEALING AGAINST ALL ODDS

AVITAL MILLER

FOREWORD BY FORBES RILEY

Dear Ashley,
You have a
beautiful life!
Joy to you,
Avital

APG Publishing

Seal Rock, OR

Published by: APG Publishing
PO Box 476
Seal Rock, OR 97376
apgpublishing.com

Editor: Ellen Kleiner
Cover Design: Cathleen Elliott
Book design: Janice St. Marie
Book formatting: Phillip Gessert

First Edition, April 2018
Copyright © 2018 by Avital Miller

The content in this book is provided for educational and informational purposes only and is not intended as a substitute for medical advice, diagnosis, treatment, or prescribing. Readers are encouraged to consult their physician on all health matters. In the event you or others use any of the information or other contents of this book, the author, contributors, and publisher assume no responsibility for the direct or indirect consequences. Some people's names have been changed to protect their privacy. The author, contributors, and publisher assume no responsibility for errors, omissions, or inconsistencies. Any slights of people or organizations are unintentional. The author does not endorse every statement, treatment, or diagnostic approach contained in this book.

Printed in the United States of America

Publisher's Cataloging-in-Publication Data
Miller, Avital, author.

Healing happens: stories of healing against all odds / Avital Miller; foreword by Forbes Riley.

ISBN: 978-0-9996785-2-7 (print) | 978-0-9996785-3-4 (eBook) | LCCN: 2017918697

Subjects: LCSH: Healing. | Alternative medicine. | Holistic medicine. | Naturopathy. | Healing–Psychological aspects. | Chronic diseases–Treatment. | Chronic diseases–Alternative treatment. | Critically ill–Treatment. | Critically ill–Alternative treatment. | Terminal care. | Healing–Psychological aspects. | Mind and body therapies. | Self-care, Health. | Nutrition. | Exercise–Physiological aspects. | Well-being. | Spiritual healing. | Mental healing. | Patients' writings. | Physicians' writings. | LCGFT: Autobiographies. | BISAC: HEALTH & FITNESS / Healing. | BODY, MIND & SPIRIT / Healing / General. | MEDICAL / Healing. | SELF-HELP / Motivational & Inspirational. | BIOGRAPHY & AUTOBIOGRAPHY / Medical.

LCC: RA776.5 .M55 2018 | DDC: 613–dc23

1 3 5 7 9 10 8 6 4 2

To my mother,

who supported me in my childhood dream to write a book, always telling me to write a little each day, and whose courage to combat cancer until the last moment of her life motivated me to do this research.

This book is also dedicated to all those wishing to suffer less and live more, to discover the healing that results from feeling happy and living their purpose.

With special thanks to:

All the health and healing practitioners I interviewed for this book, for their time, support, and dedication to helping people discover the best solutions for their health;

Ellen Kleiner, for her constant patience and commitment to making every word clearly communicate a powerful message;

Cathleen Elliott, for making the most beautiful cover image to capture the essence of healing;

Janice St. Marie, for mirroring the inspiration of this book through the visible beauty of its interior design;

Phillip Gessert, for jumping in with willingness, clarity and speed to format this book;

My many friends and family who helped me address many aspects of this book while sharing the struggles and joys of publication, and my Facebook friends for answering the many polls on finding the perfect words and designs to present its message;

The many people who helped sponsor publishing this book, especially Ian Weslek; Gregg Davison, entrepreneur; Gail Lynn, owner Life Center; Sherry Osmun Hess, founder of Legendary Spice; and Gary Rahman;

The many healers, teachers, and mentors who have believed in me, inspired me, and helped me heal so I could share this gift with others;

And to all types of healing practitioners, thank you for offering so much of your time and heart to help people realize their dreams with a healthy, happy body.

Contents

Foreword

One of the problems with health is that we only seem to be aware of it when it is failing, such as getting a cold, a broken bone, or a debilitating disease. Unaccustomed to determining how healthy we generally are, we can be caught off guard by some dire diagnosis. For instance, I am a health and fitness expert known for inspiring millions but last December I suddenly found myself in a hospital bed facing a potential diagnosis of stomach cancer. Fortunately it turned out to instead be a severe ulcer from stress, but for a week my family and I suffered the shock of having to face a potentially fatal disease. Today, I am on a quest to better understand personal health, wealth, and happiness and help others do the same.

When I first heard about Avital's healing programs, I was inspired to know more. I discovered she is an authentically joyful woman possessing wisdom beyond her years, an uplifting spirit, and has a unique ability to touch people's hearts. As someone who graduated college with two degrees (political science and communications) in only three years, I am a fan of commitment, education, and dedication. I was impressed that Avital was also a double major and graduated from a top university with both engineering and dance degrees then got a job as a program manager at Microsoft before becoming a yoga and fitness teacher trainer. She has spoken, danced, and sung for thousands of people worldwide; lived in a spiritual community for seven years; and translated what she learned from years of meditating into information anyone can understand. She is an ideal and much-needed healer for today's world.

Healing Happens not only gives an account of Avital's personal triumph over disease against all odds but also includes stories by seventeen other health and healing experts about their own or their clients' experiences overcoming diseases. I believe people are the sum of the obstacles they have overcome. Personally, growing up in the time of fast food, baloney sandwiches on white bread, and sugary breakfast cereals, I was initially blinded to good nutrition, causing me to have challenges with my weight. While I was in high school, my dad had a work accident that landed him in the hospital for almost three years, undergoing fifteen surgeries. I understood what the words *broke, lonely*, and *scared* meant. My loving parents sacrificed a lot so my sister and I wouldn't suffer, then both died of cancer at age seventy. But don't feel bad for me, because those trials helped shape my attitudes and my life mission to teach that life happens *for* you not *to* you!

Today, I am affectionately called the $2 Billion Host as I've generated product sales of millions, launched hit infomercials, and was there at the beginning of Home Shopping TV. I enjoy life as an entrepreneur, a sought-after female keynote speaker, a creator of the handheld fitness sensation SpinGym, and an inductee into the National Fitness Hall of Fame. I campaign for wellness in corporate America, offering portable and affordable solutions, and better nutrition in hospitals. With more than 2 million SpinGyms sold, I have developed a platform beyond fitness that positively addresses obesity, physical challenges, and veterans' and seniors' issues.

Avital, as a role model and champion, inspires us with her glowing inner guidance and fearless pursuit to overcome any obstacles. She was held back in elementary school for poor writing skills but today is a blogger and author. She was told she couldn't sing but joined a choir and has performed solo. She overcame an abusive marriage, a warning that moving out of her spiritual community would be "falling off the spiritual path," and a diagnosis of Hashimoto's and hypothyroidism to ultimately achieve healing. Her life represents a one-woman campaign against "you'll never."

Healing Happens is a ticket to overcoming discouragement, despondency, and despair resulting from a debilitating illness or a disease diagnosed as terminal. Worldwide, over 14 million people a year are diagnosed with cancer, one of the top three causes of death. Approximately 39.6 percent of men and women in the United States, or nearly half the population, are diagnosed with cancer at some point during their lives.[1] This book recounts stories of people who have had cancer or another deadly disease, experienced chronic pain for many years, or have been told they had only a few weeks or months to live yet today live healthy and happy lives. Their inspiring stories provide hope and motivation to others with similar diseases or conditions to persevere in their healing despite the limitations with which they have been branded.

The health experts interviewed for this book have not only in many cases healed themselves but also repeated those results for others, using a variety of techniques and methods. While their techniques and methods may not work for everyone, it can put a positive spin on a painful prognosis. Many of the procedures and practices suggested by the health practitioners interviewed—ranging from fun dietary changes to easy breathing exercises, short meditations, and shifts in perspective—can be done anywhere, on your own, in just a few minutes. The book covers over twenty different diseases and physical conditions, yet the approaches can also be applied to sustain overall wellness.

Imagine in the future, despite having been told you have a fatal disease or incurable condition, being able through these techniques to see your son or daughter walk down the aisle at their wedding, to play with your grandchildren, become a successful entrepreneur, travel, or just enjoy life pain free. *Healing Happens* aims to help you become more physically, mentally, and spiritually fit; face obstacles with your head held high; open your eyes to new healing possibilities; and become more hopeful about your potential for living a healthy, happy life.

—Forbes Riley
Creator/CEO SpinGym, motivational speaker, author,
and visionary behind the Forbes Factor

Message from the Author

I magine being told that you have only a short time to live or you have a chronic condition that you will have to put up with despite discomfort and a devastating impact on your livelihood. Alternatively, what if you or a loved one *has* received such a message. Must you or they be resigned to such a fate? At a time when the costs of medical care are high and the risk of side effects from medicine are great, people need to know that there are more ways to remain alive and healthy than are commonly followed, ranging from dietary changes to meditation to alternative medical approaches.

Learning about alternative healing methods is especially important today, given the fact that an estimated 128,000 Americans die each year as a result of taking medications as prescribed; that is more than twice as many as those who are killed in car accidents every day.[1] The cost of treating adverse drug reactions is more than $136 billion annually, greater than the total cost of cardiovascular or diabetic care.[2] Moreover, each year 440,000 patients in the United States who go to hospitals for care suffer some type of preventable harm there that contributes to their deaths, making medical errors the third leading cause of death in America, after heart disease and cancer.[3] Similar findings exist in other countries.

After coming across nearly two hundred stories of so-called miracle healings occurring in response to the application of natural healing modalities, I felt that those stories would offer important information, as well as valuable inspiration, to many people suffering from a variety of diseases. For example, Brooke Goldner, MD, thought she was going to live a short life and never be able to have children, due to lupus. Today, she has two healthy boys and has tested negative for lupus for thirteen years. The only change she made was her diet.

In 2000, Tryshe Dhevney was expected to die within a year from hepatitis C. She soon started chanting prolonged tones while playing singing bowls for the fun of it. Three months later the doctors were shocked to find no traces of hepatitis C. Today, she travels all over the United States with a large fleet of crystal bowls to help others heal.

In 2006, Maureen Belle's doctor claimed she had only six to eight weeks to live due to stage 4 non-Hodgkin's lymphoma. About three months later she weighed eighty-five pounds, was bedridden with oxygen tubes and morphine patches in hospice care, and was expected to die soon thereafter. Today she is alive, well, and sharing what she learned on her healing journey. All she did was change her perspective.

Many such miracle healing stories and alternative healing approaches are presented in *Healing Happens*. They offer hope to people suffering from such conditions as cancer, diabetes, stroke, chronic pain, chronic fatigue, ADHD, obesity, allergies, blindness, Lyme disease, Hashimoto's, hypothyroidism, multiple sclerosis, bipolar disorder, lupus, cerebral palsy, fibromyalgia, anxiety, parasites, hepatitis C, bird flu, and non-Hodgkin's lymphoma. They show how, through attitude, awareness, willpower, belief, food, sound, light, body movements, or energy therapy, people have healed despite grim prognoses.

This book shares interviews with health and healing experts like Bernie Siegel, MD, Brooke Goldner, MD, Meir Schneider, Coach Ruben, Michael Platt, MD, Nicole DeAvilla, and K. P. Stoller, MD, who repeatedly have achieved impressive healing results for themselves and others through the knowledge gleaned from their own experiences, studies, and the latest scientific research. Their medical backgrounds include study of both Eastern and Western healing modalities, as well as vast experience treating people with many different diseases. They make us aware that there are more possibilities for healing than are commonly known and help us discover the best ways to regain power over our own health and healing. And their stories need to be sung so that more people can have hope for healing and a road map to a more fulfilling and joyful life.

Not only does this book offer inspirational stories showing us how to defy the odds of a grim medical prognosis, it also provides simple techniques we can use on ourselves, sometimes in a couple minutes, as well as advice to initiate increased health and happiness. Such information includes delicious healthy foods to add to our diets, physical conditioning exercises, herbal treatments, easy breathing exercises, short meditations, and fun activities.

Although each chapter subtitle specifies one or more diseases or conditions, the chapters themselves invite the reader to look beyond diagnoses to understand the many paths to healing. Throughout, the formative question to ask is: "What helps a person heal when the usual protocol for their diagnosis does not?" Another question you might ask is: "What does true healing mean in each story and what does it mean to me?" In doing so, you may find that the healing modalities discussed in each chapter are just as applicable, if not more so, to other health challenges. You may also discover that remedies for any one condition can significantly increase overall wellness in body, mind, or spirit.

This focus on natural healing modalities was inspired by my own healing journey. I was an ambitious twenty-seven-year-old yoga and fitness expert who was diagnosed with an autoimmune disorder called Hashimoto's and hypothyroidism, was put on a high dosage of medication, and told that was it for life without being given any advice on how to actually heal. As a result of my own research and experimentation, the doctors tapered me off the medication and I started leading programs around the world to share how others can heal naturally. During that time, I met people who had been told they would die in a few months or even a few hours yet years later were completely healthy. Such encounters convinced me to help increase people's potential for healing by informing them about these victories.

In *Healing Happens*, interviews with seventeen different types of health and healing experts emphasize that there are many paths to healing. It is important to choose one that inspires you and that you believe in. Researchers like Bruce H. Lipton, PhD, show that belief in a healing protocol is one of the most important contributing factors to its success in healing.

This book suggests that so-called miracle healings no longer seem like miracles when we see them persistently repeated; it shows where risks lie in the conventional Western medicine route; it makes clear how common the side effects of medications are; it explains how many doctors focus on treating symptoms rather than healing causes; it exposes the questionable reliability of some medical research; and it illuminates how much our non-physical conditions affect our physical conditions.

We all have the potential to overcome limitations that others place on us. If a doctor gives us a prognosis we don't like, we can listen to the diagnosis yet not accept the prognosis as inevitable. The role of doctors is to heal, not tell us when we are going to die. Fatal pronouncements do not have to be our fate. *Healing Happens* offers inspiration and alternative solutions to health problems in order to open doors that readers may have never thought possible.

PART I

My Introduction to Healing

From Medication to Meditation
Healing Hashimoto's and Hypothyroidism

"There is in each of us a special song to be sung."

—Swami Kriyananda

At age twenty-five, after being a program manager at Microsoft, I began a new career in yoga and fitness. In Santa Barbara, California, I was the main instructor for 24 Hour Fitness. I also was a yoga and fitness director, teacher trainer, and business owner. There was a big poster of me at Lululemon, where they called me their most popular instructor. I taught twenty-five to thirty classes a week, rarely missing one, and always found the strength and determination to be present for my students. I was known as the "Energizer Bunny" due to the seemingly endless reserve of energy I had at my disposal to keep up with these many activities.

A year and a half into my career, in the fall of 2005, I traveled to Switzerland and then Israel for my sister's wedding. While I was hiking down the Matterhorn in Switzerland, my knee all of a sudden gave out and I fell. Fortunately, there was a cable car I could ride to the bottom, but I had to stay off my feet for the rest of my trip in Switzerland. Then in Israel I had headaches and such low energy that I needed naps for the first time in my life.

Several months later, while leading a spinning class, I felt nauseous, light-headed, physically weak, and, oddly, like I had wet my underpants. When I went to the bathroom, I realized it was blood and became concerned since it was not the time of month for that to be happening. Nevertheless, I stuffed toilet paper in my underwear, took a deep breath, and returned to the studio determined to finish the class. But as I became weaker and my face got whiter my students urged me to end the class early and go to the hospital, so I drove myself there. At the hospital, the doctor could not determine a diagnosis so she ran blood tests and sent me home. Even though I got better after several days, I was scared to go back to teach spinning classes and had others substitute for me. After a week, the doctor explained my blood test results all looked good except for the thyroid number. Since it was only slightly off and I was so young, she thought that should not be an issue.

Shortly afterward I caught a cold and had a persistent fever. At the time, I was in a business development course to take my business to the next level, and everyone was amazed that despite how sick I was I kept up with all the classes.

A month later I still had the fever; my hair was falling out more than normal; I had extra wax in my ears; I was experiencing abnormal digestion, fatigue, and headaches; and I sometimes could not see well. It seemed like my body was becoming progressively weaker, and I worried that I would soon be out of the job. Sometimes at night I could feel my heart pounding against the bed and needed to adjust my position so I could breathe. Other times I could feel pain in parts of my body where I had never felt it before. I would wake up with swollen eyelids, my ankles would swell on airline flights, and I was cold all the time. I was concerned about how I, who had always felt invincible, could suddenly become so sick. I wondered if I would just keep getting worse until I died.

Since the doctor had not been able to give me a diagnosis and treatment plan, I did some research online. With so many diseases having similar symptoms, I started to fear I could have numerous fatal diseases. Eventually, I came across an autoimmune disease that seemed to best reflect my symptoms—Hashimoto's thyroiditis. Traditionally described as the body attacking the thyroid gland, doctors believed Hashimoto's compromises the thyroid gland's ability to function and leads to hypothyroidism. Hypothyroidism is a condition where the body does not produce sufficient thyroid hormone to function well. The most common symptoms are fatigue, depressive moods, and weight gain. I asked one of my doctors to test my level of thyroid peroxidase antibodies (TPO ab). He confirmed the diagnosis of Hashimoto's and prescribed thyroid hormone.

I had a sense of relief when I received my diagnosis because then I could have a clear direction on what actions to take to feel better. My doctors advised me that Hashimoto's was a lifelong disease and I would be on medication for life. I believed my doctors and decided if it was for life I would do my best with it. I trusted that if it was meant to be a part of my life, I would accomplish what I was meant to accomplish. That doesn't mean that I liked having a disease or being on medication, but I held a vision of a brighter future without this hindrance. I had big dreams of helping people around the world live a happy and healthy life. I felt the symptoms I was experiencing could get in the way of those dreams so I assumed they would not last. That mindset helped me relax. The other thought that came to mind soon after my diagnosis was that perhaps the diseases had occurred to offer me wisdom to help others heal from Hashimoto's and hypothyroidism.

A few months later one of my middle-aged yoga students complained about her issues with hypothyroidism and ended with saying, "You probably can't relate to any of this. You are too young." Unfortunately, I could now easily relate to the many people, potentially 60 million in the United States alone, with thyroid disorders.[1]

As for the thyroid hormone I had been prescribed, I had a difficult experience with it. I had been told that women over forty on this medication were at high risk of osteoporosis and that the thyroid gland could die out in time and need to be removed. I squirmed each time I took it, partly because I did not like being on allopathic medicine but also because it was made from pig, which seemed repulsive to me, having kept kosher all my life and aspiring to become a vegetarian. Discovering the right types and dosages of other thyroid medications was also problematic, the many adjustments making it hard to teach my classes. As well, each doctor I saw added more tests to the thyroid panel—T3, T4, Free T3, Free T4, TSH, TPO Ab, Free Thyroxine—and there was also a full panel of blood tests for vitamin levels, cholesterol, iron, and white blood cell count. Ultimately, I ended up taking 150 mcg of Synthroid for T4 and 10 mcg of Cytomel for T3 every day. The doctor was worried that I would be allergic to the dye in the higher dosage pills, so instead prescribed three white 50 mcg Synthroid pills and two 5 mcg Cytomel pills per day. That amounted to five pills a day plus a handful of supplements!

I remained uncertain about the overall effectiveness of this regimen. If I didn't take the pills at the same time every morning and an hour before eating, I noticed subtle differences in my energy and ability to think during the day. The theory that was explained to me for taking thyroid hormone for Hashimoto's was to stop the thyroid gland from producing the hormone. That would cause the antibodies to stop noticing the gland and thus the body to stop attacking the gland, potentially resulting in the gland eventually dying. I was skeptical of this theory first because it seemed like a workaround with negative side effects rather than a solution that heals the initial reason for having this issue. Second, because the level of antibodies in my body nearly tripled after three years of having my thyroid hormone level balanced on medication.

Also I didn't feel well on this regimen, so the doctors tested for everything else under the sun, including allergies, parasites, adrenal gland function, cortisone layers, metal poisoning, uric acid, heart murmur, and vitamin levels. They advised me to go on three different elimination diets and to set up a petri dish to test for mold in my home. During those many visits to doctors' offices I often felt sicker the longer I was there waiting and being poked by needles to run so many tests.

I ended up with a list of foods I was allergic to, including what had been my staple diet in Switzerland, chocolate and bread, which explained my fatigue in Israel. The doctors also added to the list of diagnoses hypoglycemic, borderline anemic, low levels of vitamins and protein, and slight heart murmur. Consequently, I was told to eat more red meat for protein, as well as oil and butter to help balance my hormones, and to take daily supplements.

By this time I was $8,000 in debt from out-of-pocket medical expenses and discouraged about my prognosis for the future.

Then three experiences ignited a spark of hope that I might not have to suffer my whole life from the conditions diagnosed by my doctor. The first experience was while laying on a massage table with an energy healer working on me. She calmly and confidently whispered in my ear, "Just because your mom has hypothyroidism does not mean you have to have it." That to me meant disease is not dictated by heredity. The second experience occurred when I went to an acupuncturist at a local college for pain in my knee. I saw a student practitioner there eating a weird vegetable meal that she claimed had helped her heal from hypothyroidism, alerting me to the possibility of healing the disease through diet. The third experience was reading about how when Oprah discovered she had hypothyroidism she took a month off and cured herself. I later read that may not be true, but at the time it made me hopeful that I could heal too.

Now even more determined to focus on healing, I continued to research Hashimoto's and hypothyroidism online and in books; went to an endocrinologist, holistic doctors, Ayurvedic doctors, acupuncturists, naturopaths, and energy healers; and even studied one-on-one with an Ayurvedic doctor in India for two months. In addition, I began to pay more attention to all aspects of my lifestyle. Even though as a yoga and fitness professional I knew a lot about living a healthy lifestyle, I realized there was more to learn. I had to be especially particular about diet because the suggested diet for people with Hashimoto's was different from that for people with hypothyroidism. I also had to be careful about habits, such as sleeping at a particular time of night, avoiding environmental toxins, and not over-exercising.

What I learned while dealing with these various aspects of health opened my eyes to things I had not known and changed my perspective. I discovered research about how our health may be undermined by the way food is produced and packaged, by specific products, and by the quality of water we drink. I came across articles revealing potential corruption in the medical industry, particularly where research is funded and conducted by the people or companies that profit from the results.[2] I learned counterintuitive statistics such as that countries with the highest rates of osteoporosis are where people drink the most milk, whereas countries with the lowest rates of osteoporosis are where people consume the least amount of milk.[3] I became aware that research shows our bodies are only 7 percent protein. Therefore, I concluded we may be eating more meat than necessary, especially considering protein is easier for the body to absorb from dark leafy greens, and those greens have high amounts of protein. For example, 60 percent of the calories from kale are protein.[4]

I also learned that chemicals in many of the cleaning, hair, and skin products we use can be harmful to us, as are many of the chemicals and other substances in our environment.[5] For instance, the air in some cities contains toxic substances from chemtrails or chemicals used to treat and fertilize nonorganic farms. Furthermore, city water is often treated with chlorine and fluorine, which have been shown to cause hypothyroidism.[6] That explains why I was getting tired and delirious after swimming in pool water treated with chlorine. It was hard to find bottled water companies that stated the ingredients contained in their "drinking" water, so I switched to drinking distilled water. Then I found out that drinking distilled water is not a good idea because it can continually detox the body. Today I have a water machine that both purifies the water of chlorine, fluorine, heavy metals, and pesticides and produces hydrogen-enriched alkalized water.

I learned a lot more about body dynamics related to water and health. For instance, it has been shown that hydrogen has therapeutic potential for essentially every organ of the body and for 150 different diseases.[7] A higher level of alkalinity is known to overcome fatigue, depression, poor digestion, candida, weight retention, diabetes, cancer, and cellular degeneration. Naturally alkaline rich foods are dark leafy greens, fruits, and other vegetables.[8] An easy trick for alkalizing water is to squeeze lemon juice into it; it is also advantageous, when possible, to use well water as its treatment can be controlled. Since our bodies are made mostly of water,[9] and it is important that what we put into them matches their natural state, eating more raw and hydrated foods and avoiding overcooked and processed foods is beneficial to health. When dehydrated food enters our bodies, it leaches water out of our cells, which then seem like foreign substances; the body subsequently attacks these cells to get rid of them, as I learned from one of my doctors who was also an acupuncturist. Thus an autoimmune disorder is the body attacking not itself but rather what seems foreign to it. Anthony William, also known as the Medical Medium, even suggests that Hashimoto's is the result of the body trying to remove Epstein–Barr virus from the thyroid gland, a premise that medical research has not yet uncovered.[10]

Visits with my acupuncturist/MD further enlightened me about the risks associated with traditional medicine, as well as the benefits of dietary changes. He asked me, "Do you know that more people die under the knife of a doctor than not? Do you know doctors die faster than anyone else?" While proof of such statements is hard to find, it is estimated that around 128,000 people die each year from taking medications as prescribed and about 440,000 patients a year who go to the hospital for care suffer some type of preventable harm that contributes to their deaths.[11] My acupuncturist/MD also changed my perspective on the effects of diet on health through graphic illustrations. He picked up a book and asked me how old I thought the man on the cover was. I guessed thirty. The man was fifty! Then he grabbed another book and asked me how old its author looked. I answered, "Fifty?" He replied, "Eighty." Those authors had eaten primarily a superfood diet of raw smoothies with all sorts of rich greens and fruits.

During this time I did my best to follow the doctor's orders and include meat in one or two meals a day, despite my lifelong dream of becoming a vegetarian. But I also started adding superfoods to my diet, making smoothies and interesting, colorful vegetable dishes. Soon I could taste fruits and vegetables like I never had before, which was wonderful.

The acupuncturist/MD also did more extensive blood tests than other doctors. He looked at my blood cells under a microscope projected on a screen, noting that each ring in the cells, like those in a tree trunk, represented how deeply embedded an issue was, while the patterning in each ring indicated the prevalent disease. He determined my thyroid problem was more of a surface issue, while my digestive problems were more ingrained, likely originating in childhood. These observations made me believe more in my potential to heal my thyroid.

Additionally, he made me aware of how my emotions related to my organs. After just two weeks of adding superfoods to my diet, I mentioned how I had not become angry about something that normally would have upset me. He responded, "Good. That means your liver is working better." Then I shared how I had handled another challenging situation better than in the past. He replied, "Good. That means your kidneys are working better."

As the weeks passed, I tried all sorts of herbs, tinctures, and supplements; read about the emotions associated with hypothyroidism; paid more attention to my thoughts and emotions; and ended some unhealthy relationships. I also took note of the activities that made me tired and adjusted my life accordingly. Usually, it was foods I was allergic to that made me tired, and doing things I loved that made me energetic.

I even found scientific findings supporting the notion that hypothyroidism does not have to be hereditary. Bruce Lipton, a stem cell biologist and bestselling author of *The Biology of Belief*, researched the relationship between disease and genetics, called epigenetics. He discovered that a child born into a family without the cancer gene and adopted by one with the cancer gene has the same propensity to get cancer as any natural child in that family, suggesting that cancer may be caused by perceptions, beliefs, and attitudes. I was instantly intrigued by the idea that making one's thoughts more positive than the environment might prevent a person from experiencing the same illnesses as others in that environment.

Similarly, I came to believe that the body wants to heal itself. Treating it in a more loving way, while not dwelling on harmful thoughts about its deficiencies, can support healing. For example, an astrologer told me not to think of my Hashimoto's in warlike terms, as if I were battling it, lest I encourage even more "war" to manifest internally.

After researching and trying different healing modalities, I realized that entertaining so many different approaches could itself be stressful. So one morning, as I was getting ready to take my daily dosage of a disgusting-tasting tincture, I decided that to avoid unnecessary stress it was time to follow only the healing practices I enjoyed and those I intuited would be helpful. A few months after implementing my new habits, I felt more balanced, freed of so many emotional and physical ups and downs. Disease had stopped being the center of my attention, and I was enjoying life again.

I took another big leap forward by leaving my successful career in Santa Barbara and my marriage to move into a spiritual community and to accept a job as a full-time fitness director in the Bay Area. The environment of the spiritual community, which had been founded by Swami Kriyananda, a direct disciple of the yoga guru Paramhansa Yogananda, helped me meditate regularly for longer periods of time. I also did so with a higher power in mind, that we often call God, Source, or the Divine. After a month of living in the spiritual community, I lost my craving for meat and realized my dream of becoming a vegetarian. Previously, I had only been able to adhere to such a diet for brief periods of time, perhaps because my body wasn't ready and I didn't have a replacement diet that I loved; it is hard to say whether I was able to finally stay on a vegetarian diet because meditation made my body crave lighter foods or because I had added so many vegetables to my diet that I was getting enough nutrients without meat. Whatever the reason, as a result of this new diet my body felt more energetic and flexible.

After a few months of meditating, I started to have headaches—my body's longtime default symptom anytime something was off. I felt tired yet hyper; my body was heating up easily; and I had trouble sleeping. Through the spiritual community, I connected with a naturopathic doctor, Connie Hernandez, ND, and went to see her. Following more blood and thyroid tests, she found that my iron level was low, which accounted for the fatigue; yet my thyroid level was too high, which explained everything else. As a result, she lowered my dosage of thyroid medication, advised me about supplements, and suggested creative activities for healing. One activity was to walk barefoot on grass in the morning while the dew was still on the land to help ground me. I was excited about connecting with the dew since that is part of the translation of my name in Hebrew, and I thought that getting in touch with the earth would help me align with the biochemistry of my body. She also advised wearing turquoise shawls around my neck would have a cooling and healing effect, as the color matches the vibration of the throat chakra. That thrilled me because I loved the color turquoise and enjoyed dressing up with a shawl.

About this time I also became aware that many practitioners viewed focusing on the throat chakra as important in healing hypothyroidism since the disease is in the area of the throat. The throat chakra has to do with communication, and although I communicated a lot while teaching so many classes, I needed to better communicate my deeper feelings in personal relationships. Later, an Ayurvedic doctor in California encouraged me to learn to communicate my "sweet song," an intimate, authentic means of calmly communicating deeper emotions in a way that is received well by others—a skill useful both for personal healing and for the well-being of others in the world. As I gained a better understanding of myself and my emotions, it became easier to communicate my "sweet song," increasing my confidence in being able to enhance my own and others' health.

I realized not only is it important for our own healing to share our song, but also for the world. Upon discovering that many agents that cause hypothyroidism and other diseases are from our environment, water, food, and household products, I saw the importance of using our voice to let people know how our health has been impacted. My hope has been that this inspires more businesses to make better decisions on how they operate to support not only their own growth but also the health of the world.

Within a month of following Dr. Hernandez's advice, including lowering my dosage of medication, I felt better. After another month I again felt ill, and she again determined that I was taking too much medication. She lowered my dosage, which made me feel better. But then a couple months later the same thing occurred. Over the next four years the pattern of not feeling well and then lowering my dosage continued to repeat itself.

All the while, I was discovering increasingly more about my conditions and possible treatments. To help me further reduce my intake of medication, one of my doctors advised me to switch the dosage every other day between a higher and lower amount.

My Ayurvedic doctor in California could assess how my thyroid was doing by reading my pulse. She gave me some powerful herbal teas to strengthen my thyroid, aid digestion, and balance my moods. Having left a job that had afforded me insurance and a good income to move to the spiritual community's center in the foothills of the Sierra Nevadas in Northern

California, and having been denied insurance while trying to get it on my own, I figured I might as well pursue healing paths that costed less and felt less invasive. Since that Ayurvedic doctor lived an hour away yet could read my pulse intuitively, I started to work with her over the phone. Then I realized that I too was tuning into how much medication I needed. I requested to alter my dosage myself rather than having an appointment every one to two months and she agreed. Some days I forgot to take the medication, while other days when I felt my energy drop or got a headache I took extra medication. For about a year after I stopped needing any medication, I still carried my medication in a little yellow plastic candy case that had come out of a piñata at a party until I summoned the courage to throw the case and medication away.

Ultimately, it is hard to say exactly what actions, treatments, or practices resulted in my healing. Determining this is like trying to figure out how a group of novice rowers struggling to propel a boat across a big lake, who then hire a trainer to teach them effective rowing techniques and are subsequently subjected to a strong gust of wind, are finally able to sail swiftly across the lake. Was this outcome propelled by their determination, techniques taught by the trainer, or the gust of wind? Regarding my healing, all I know is that after making significant changes to my diet, lifestyle, relationships, and environment I felt steady. As I increased my time spent in meditation, I had managed to wean myself from the thyroid medicine, shifting from medication to meditation.

Among the more than three thousand scientific studies exploring the benefits of meditation, my favorite is on the impact of meditation on biological age. People who had been practicing meditation for less than five years were found to be physiologically up to *five* years younger than their chronological age as determined by lower blood pressure and better near-point vision and auditory discrimination. People who had been practicing meditation for more than five years were found to be physiologically *twelve* years younger than their chronological age.[12]

Although I prefer natural healing methods, I am grateful for the medication's support when I have had trouble functioning. And while my health is not always perfect, I am grateful for moments of not feeling entirely well because they teach me a way to improve my life. Rather than blame our-selves for disease, I feel we can see it as a sign that we are ready for growth.

I saw another gift in my health struggles when the spiritual community published a book of Paramhansa Yogananda's writings entitled *How to Achieve Glowing Health and Vitality* that mirrored my experience in tending to the physical, energetic, mental, emotional, and spiritual layers of healing. This event triggered a memory of the desire I had had, upon first receiving my diagnosis, to help others heal. As sales and marketing director of the publishing company, I was tasked with the job of promoting its books, but I gave this one extra attention and taught its principles around the world. In 2015, I moved out of the spiritual community to fully dedicate myself to helping others with all layers of healing in a more universal way. As I con-tinue to travel, study, and grow, my understanding of healing continually evolves, as it can for all of us if we stay open to it.

WISDOM TO REMEMBER

1. Don't Listen to Everything

Don't automatically accept as fact everything doctors tell you. We are all used to the refrain "Listen to your doctor." But I feel doctors are meant to help us heal, not decide how a condition will affect our lives in the future or when we are going to die. My doctors did not tell me I could get off medication, and yet I did. I have also come across people living well beyond the time their doctors predicted they would die. In addition, I learned that much of the food we eat, air we breathe, and many products we put on our bodies are not as safe as we may be told. Our bodies have a greater potential to heal from chronic conditions than we may realize, so it is important to keep an open mind and look for open doors.

2. Focus on Your Reason to Live

Aids to my healing were focusing on why I wanted to live and the dreams I wanted to accomplish. While I didn't like having challenges with my health I trusted everything would work out. I discovered doing what I loved helped distract me from pain and gave me the energy to move forward.

3. Do What You Can Do

Since the various layers of healing—physical, energetic, mental, emotional, and spiritual—are interconnected, do what you can and like to do in order to easily and enjoyably effect positive change. For example, if you can't alter your emotions to feel good, change your diet; and as your body heals, your emotions may become more positive. If you can't change your eating habits, meditate; the calmness it brings will likely shift the types of food you crave to match that state of inner peace.

4. Ask "What Is the Gift?"

I do not believe disease comes to us as a divine retribution for anything we have done wrong. When you have a chronic condition or face a big medical challenge you can feel happier if you can identify the gifts in the situation. For instance, my health challenges led to a new career, about which I am passionate; taught me how powerful I am; resulted in more supportive and inspiring relationships; and helped me learn a lot about the body, the mind, emotions, and spirit that I can use to help others live more fulfilling lives.

WHAT YOU CAN DO

- Experiment with a healthier diet and find fun replacements for foods you are allergic to or that do not support your well-being.

- Choose a hydrated diet with more raw and less processed and over-cooked foods.

- Eat a colorful, alkaline-rich assortment of fruits, vegetables, and dark leafy greens.

- Drink purified, alkalized water. An easy way to alkalize water is to add lemon. For best results, squeeze a lemon into a cup of warm water in the mornings and drink.

- Replace household products containing harmful chemicals with natural alternatives. If you decide to make just one change, replace your dryer sheets.

- Become aware of when your energy level, thoughts, and emotions are down, and add or eliminate activities accordingly to shift to a more positive and energetic state.

- If you have a meditation or spiritual practice, maintain it; if not, sit quietly or walk alone in nature for frequent breaks from external distractions and to gain new perspectives.

- Discover your authentic, intimate voice, your "sweet song," and share it.

PART II

Nutrition and Healing

CHAPTER 2

Shifting from Surviving to Thriving
Reversing Diabetes

With
Ruben J. Guzman, MPH, ACLM

"Look deep into nature, and then you will understand everything better."

—Albert Einstein

When a friend recommended I speak to Ruben J. Guzman, known as Coach Ruben, little did I know how much he would inspire me with his stories and wisdom. The author of *Evolving Health: Maximize Your Energy Using the Wisdom of Science and Divine Design*, Coach Ruben is also a speaker, sports and healthy lifestyle coach, and member of the American College of Lifestyle Medicine. He has been in the health industry for over forty years, changing people's lives by teaching them life-promoting behavior so they not only survive but thrive.

Coach Ruben, would you tell us about what you do.

I wear several hats. I'm kind of a renaissance man. When it comes to health, I empower people to fundamentally change from a sympathetic nervous system state of survival, in which their body exhibits chronic disease and depleted energy, to a parasympathetic nervous system state so that their body can heal itself. This is a different concept from what I was taught in medical school. It's about shifting the wiring and energy state of how the body functions because the body wants to heal and thrive.

Do you have any stories that illustrate such a shift in somebody, comparing what would typically happen in a situation handled by the medical industry and the success you were able to achieve?

Certainly. One of my favorite stories is about Angela. I met her when she was fifteen years old and I was her swimming coach. I coached swimmers professionally for thirty years, and she was one of my outstanding swimmers.

When we first met, she was disillusioned, unhappy, and frustrated. Her previous coaches had told her that because she had gotten heavy she was never going to make it at the big-time level. But she started swimming with me, and within a short time I was able to see her potential. I told her, "I see what's possible for you. If you're willing to be coachable, we can get somewhere in this sport. I really believe in you." That's what she needed—somebody to believe in her. As a result, six months later she qualified within the top 1 percent of championship swimmers in the United States.

By the time she finished swimming with me, in her senior year of high school, she ended up with a full scholarship in swimming and academics to an excellent university. In university, once again, she was an outstanding student and an accomplished athlete. As a collegiate athlete she trained two to two and a half hours a day. But then she graduated.

In the background for her were her family's dietary patterns. Her father was diabetic, and her mother had a stroke shortly after Angela graduated from college. Angela had a background of eating a particular way. By the time she was twenty-three, she noticed that her blood sugar was going up over 100. When she was twenty-five, she was diagnosed with type 2 diabetes and put on insulin injections to manage her blood sugar. Now this is a very bright, capable, and intelligent woman who read the literature and worked with her doctors, but the complications increased.

By the time she was thirty-two, in 2012, she had a long list of complications, including peripheral neuropathy. Her vision was deteriorating. She had blood pressure problems, cholesterol issues, and heart palpitations. She couldn't even swim anymore because it was too painful.

Her doctor told her, "Your A1C is 10 percent, and your blood sugar is over 200, which is double what it should be. We're going to have to put you on another medication. I don't know what else we can do." She began looking at her blood sugar values and interpreting them. She realized that her kidneys were starting to fail, that within a short time she was going to have to be on dialysis, and that if things continued the way they were going she would probably not live much longer.

Out of desperation Angela called me and said, "Ruben, I've looked at everything, and I don't know what to do anymore. I'm wondering if you can help me."

I responded, "Angela, we're going to beat this diabetes if it's the last thing we do. But are you willing to be as coachable as you were when you swam with me? It's going to take that."

She replied, "Yes, I am."

So we went to work. I had her read *Dr. Neal Barnard's Program for Reversing Diabetes*, the best material available on a nutritional approach to diabetes. I told her to set up an appointment with her doctor. On September 10, 2012, we measured her blood sugar: it was 196, and her A1C was 10 percent. We started measuring her blood glucose level three times a day, and she followed the program to the letter.

Four days later her blood sugar was down to 123, so she didn't have to take an injection—for the first time in seven years! Seven days later her blood sugar was down to 93; this was the first time her blood sugar was under 100 in nine years! Ten days after that her blood sugar was down to 72, which is below the normal range. I worked with her doctor, and we instituted a protocol to reduce medications and get her off them gradually so that she would not become hypoglycemic with the low blood sugar.

Although we focused only on nutritional and stress management work, she continued to make progress. Ten months later Angela was off all medications. The doctor could hardly believe it, at which point we gave him a copy of Barnard's book. The doctor exclaimed, "This is phenomenal. You don't need medications, and you don't need to see me anymore." She hasn't had to have an injection since, and it's been almost four years.

The most important thing to me was that when Angela called me she was wondering who to bequeath her belongings and life insurance policy to because she knew she was probably not going to be alive more than a few years yet she had developed a new lease on life, literally. She is now completing a doctorate degree, which by its nature will help people avoid the challenges she faced. Isn't that fabulous?

That is! It's amazing to consider this woman's potential, the level of risk she experienced, and then the way you turned her life around—twice. I think people will be curious about the key factors involved in helping her.

Here is my basic premise for how we work as human beings. Before I went to medical school, I majored in biology at Cal Lutheran University, where my professor Dr. Mike Kolinsky explained, "Remember that all of life is either thriving or surviving at any moment in time. And that's all there is."

I raised my hand and asked, "How can that be? I don't get it." He replied, "Sit with it, Ruben. You'll figure it out."

When I was in medical school taking a course in embryology, I connected the dots, realizing, among other things, that as human beings we start off in the amazing process of creating life. Embryology is the study of the development of the human body from the moment of conception to the time when everything is there, which is usually by the end of the first trimester in utero. At a certain point all the cells look alike. Shortly after that a tube develops, called the neural tube, which becomes the central nervous system that then divides into two systems: the sympathetic and the parasympathetic. It's a two-wire electrical system just like the electrical system in your house, where there is a black wire and a white wire for any fixture. If you're building a house, you don't want to put the electrical system in last, after the sheetrock is already in. You want to put it in early. The same is true of us—that is the divine design.

The sympathetic nervous system is the black wire. This is about stress and survival. Whenever the sympathetic nervous system is triggered, we immediately react with flight, fight, or freeze, depending on how we deal with perceived threats. Then there is the parasympathetic nervous system, which is the white wire. This is about peace, pleasure, rest, digestion, fun, play, and eating. Whenever the parasympathetic nervous system is triggered, we move into a relaxed and thriving state.

Here is the fundamental truth of how we are as human beings: we operate either the sympathetic or the parasympathetic system at any moment. We can never operate both at the same time. We can go back and forth between the two, but we don't cross the wires as that would cause a short. We are either thriving or surviving. When I worked with Angela, it was amazing to understand that having diabetes and all those complications was because she was too often in a sympathetic state.

There are five major influences that determine whether we are in a sympathetic or a parasympathetic state. The first, and foremost, influence is the thoughts we think. Buddha said, "We are what we think." A lot of people believe we are what we eat, not what we think; but our thoughts are more powerful because thoughts can become things. Everything we think becomes manifested. There is a wonderful book by Napoleon Hill called *Think and Grow Rich* and also a book entitled *As a Man Thinketh* by James Allen, both of which address how we think. Even the Bible says, in Proverbs 23:7, "For as a man thinks in his heart, so is he." Because our thoughts are powerful, we need to be aware of them and manage them.

The second major influence on the state of our central nervous system is the words we speak. Words can either heal or destroy. Being aware of the words we speak is critical. If we suffer from "stinkin' thinkin'" as Zig Ziglar used to say, or from "stinkin' speakin'" as I say, then we're going to have issues. We will trigger the sympathetic nervous system, which will cause us to be in a state of survival. So it's important for us to mind our words. I love the Arabian proverb: "The words of the tongue should have three gatekeepers: Is it true? Is it kind? And is it necessary?" Sometimes we can focus on one of the three, but it's important to get all three.

The third major influence on the state of our central nervous system is the actions we take. Actions speak louder than words. This is a matter of being able to walk our talk. Author and educator Stephen Covey said, "As we make and keep commitments, even small commitments, we begin to establish an inner integrity that gives us the awareness of self-control and the courage and strength to accept more of the responsibility for our own lives. By making and keeping promises to ourselves and others, little by little, our honor becomes greater than our moods."

And keeping promises to ourselves comes before keeping promises to others.

Absolutely. The problem for many of us who are unhealthy is that we make promises to ourselves like, "I'm going to go to the gym on Monday." Our subconscious mind says, "Yeah, right. I don't believe you." Then Monday comes around, and sure enough, we sabotage ourselves yet again. It's important to recognize the power of our actions, especially in relationship to our promises.

Some people say, "I won't promise anything." That's like being a ship in a harbor and never doing anything. You're not living. If you want to live an extraordinary life, you have to make promises and keep them. That's powerful.

The fourth major influence on the state of our central nervous system is the company we keep. Show me your friends and I'll show you your future. Motivational speaker Jim Rohn taught, "You are the average of the five people you spend the most time with," and psychological research has supported this. Our inner circle of five is critical to evaluate. Are these the people we want to emulate and be like in our lives? If we have people in our inner circle who have "stinkin' thinkin'" and "stinkin' speakin'" and no integrity, we may have to do a people-ectomy. I've had to do that. I've said: "I love this person, but I cannot afford to have this person in my life because they are pulling my energy down. They are draining me, and I need to elevate who I am and what I'm committed to in my life. Therefore, I'm going to have to do a people-ectomy." Every time I've done it things worked out for the better.

I've done it, too. It's very hard to cut somebody out, especially if you love them and feel very connected with them. If you don't have a lot of options, it's even more scary. But you will notice that as soon as you decide to shift, you start moving more quickly in your desired direction—and that empty space gets filled up pretty quickly.

I couldn't agree with you more. The fifth major influence on the state of the central nervous system is the food we eat. This is surprising to a lot of people since most of us don't view food from a neurological perspective. When somebody is serving hors d'oeuvres at a party, you don't ask, "Will this affect me in the parasympathetic or sympathetic system?" But food is either life promoting or life depleting.

It's not just about whether something looks good, tastes good, and smells good. There are a lot of foods we can put in our mouths that look, taste, and smell really good, but that doesn't mean they'll promote our health and our life. Food is going to trigger either the sympathetic or the parasympathetic nervous system.

What are some foods people might not commonly think of as triggering the sympathetic nervous system?

Let's start with foods that cause inflammation. One is dairy—specifically from a cow, goat, or other mammal. Most of us don't think about how their milk affects us neurologically. We hear ads that say milk does a body good and we need milk for strong bones, but we don't think about it from the divine design perspective. Do you know, Avital, how many species of mammals there are on the planet?

How many?

There are over five thousand species of mammals. Even as a biology major I had no idea about their nursing behaviors, so I decided to ask some professors at the UC Davis School of Veterinary Medicine two important questions. The first question was: "For the last ten thousand years, as far as we can tell, how many of the over five thousand species of mammals on the planet have been routinely nursing from a different species of mammal by choice?"

They answered, "Ruben, it doesn't happen. Zero." None of the five thousand species of mammals on the planet has been routinely nursing from a different species by choice. There are exceptions, but only every now and then. No cows get nursed by humans by choice—they are enslaved. And that's how we produce our dairy. Milk is a slavery by-product.

The second question I asked the professors was: "Out of the over five thousand species of mammals on the planet, how many have been routinely nursing past infancy by choice?"

They answered, "Ruben, it doesn't happen."

Therefore, we can conclude that every species should be nursed only by their own and only during infancy. Humans' departure from this natural pattern is problematic. The consumption of dairy causes inflammation and many other complications, especially in the American population.

Another food that causes inflammation and other problems is meat, especially highly processed meat like salami, pastrami, pepperoni, and hot dogs. We will probably soon be advocating that a label be put on those food products because there is now sufficient evidence—as much evidence as we had with cigarettes—that those foods cause cancer. We're not designed to eat the meat from domesticated animals either.

The only animals that are designed to consume other animals have claws, talons, beaks or sharp canines, and no molars. Open a cat's mouth and take a good look inside: there are no molars. Dogs, same thing. We have molars, which are for grinding and mashing vegetables, plant material. So do hippopotamuses and gorillas; in fact, gorillas can eat sixty pounds of plant material a day. When people who know I'm vegetarian ask, "Where do you get your protein?" I say from spinach.

I have a study that shows the percentage of protein in various vegetables. We are mistaken in thinking that we need protein from meat.

Americans have been duped into believing media reports from the meat and dairy industries stating that we need a tremendous amount of meat or dairy protein, and that's not true. The leading deficiency in this country is not protein. We haven't had a case of protein deficiency among healthy people in over a hundred years. The leading deficiency is fiber—97 percent of the American population is deficient in fiber.

Also processed oils such as olive oil, sesame seed oil, and safflower oil cause inflammation and serious problems.

And then there are toxins that trigger the sympathetic system immediately and cause serious side effects in the body. One such toxin is refined sugar, or any derivative of refined sugar. Even the stuff that says "organic turbinado raw sugar" is processed. It's a man-made sugar; it's not divinely made. And there's a difference.

Fried foods, also toxic, are basically embalmed. Think about formaldehyde and embalming; that's what deep frying does to food.

Sodas are also very toxic because fundamentally they are saltwater solutions dressed up with sweeteners, coloring, and flavoring. Drinking soda is no different from being stranded in the ocean drinking salt water, which is not a good idea because you would get dehydrated. The British said that sailors who drank salt water from the ocean and were still alive when rescued exhibited delirium. That's where the word *delirious* comes from. Salt water dehydrates the brain, which is about 80 percent water. Sodas also dehydrate the brain. We're seeing from the research that they also contribute to Alzheimer's.

Another toxin is legal drugs. While many illegal drugs are toxic to the body, some legal drugs also have toxic side effects. Nicotine is one such drug. You can smoke cigarettes, but it's toxic. If you were to convert nicotine into a liquid and let one drop of it touch your skin, you would be dead in five seconds—It's that toxic.

Caffeine is a cousin of nicotine. In fact, the extraction process for both substances is exactly the same. In my organic chemistry class, I remember asking my professor Dr. Wiley, "So if the nicotine would kill me, what happens if I were careless and let a drop of caffeine touch my skin?" He replied, "Well, it won't quite kill you. Chances are you would get very sick." However, it could potentially kill someone who is young or old. People don't realize what they're dealing with when they drink that cup of coffee or that soda with caffeine. It's very important to recognize this. Alcohol is another legal drug with toxic side effects.

Finally there are excitotoxins—food additives—about which Dr. Russell Blaylock has written a couple books. Excitotoxins are substances like MSG, BHT, and aspartame that are added to preserve food and enhance flavor. We've noticed from neuroscience that these products overstimulate cells in the brain to the point of causing nerve death. Excitotoxins are also considered a contributing factor to the development of Alzheimer's.

All these substances that trigger the sympathetic nervous system are life depleting. They are not whole foods. They are not what I call divine food.

Divine food consists of various categories of energy foods that promote life. The first category is whole grains—like oats, millet, spelt, and barley—as opposed to processed grains.

Another category of energy food that qualifies as divine food is legumes, which are fabulous. What we've seen in the research is that the number-one food common to the longest living groups of people on the planet is legumes, such as beans, peas, and lentils. There are over two thousand varieties. That's a lot to choose from, so you can't get bored.

A third category is starchy vegetables, which have a high concentration of starch for energy. These include potatoes, sweet potatoes, and squashes.

A fourth category is antioxidants and anti-aging foods, which are important for all biochemical functions in the body. They're not fuel, but they provide a lot of the other nutrients we need, especially micronutrients. These foods include vegetables and fruits of all colors, of which there's a great variety. It's good to eat a lot of greens, especially leafy greens, as well as eggplant, squash, you name it. And you can knock yourself out eating fruits—have them all.

Nuts, seeds, and avocados are a special category. They are healthy sources of fat; but if you've got too much fat in your body and have a chronic disease or chronic condition, you'll want to reduce the amount of fat in your diet. Until you're healthy, you don't want to consume nuts, seeds, and avocados. People ask me, "Don't we need fat in our diet?" I say, "Absolutely—provided you're not wearing extra fat. If you are, burn off the extra fat first, then start including some nuts, seeds, and avocados in your diet."

So nothing from animals—no meat, no milk. No eggs?

No eggs. Eggs are pre-embryonic animals, which means they aren't even developed. They are extremely high in cholesterol and other unwanted components. Most people don't realize that cholesterol is a steroidal compound—the grandmother of all steroidal hormones, including testosterone, estrogen, progesterone, cortisol, and aldosterone.

According to our divine design, we do not require cholesterol in our diet. Any time we ingest cholesterol, the pituitary gland, the "manager" in the brain, says, "Okay, I've got this extra supply. Manufacture more downstream hormones," which are needed for the body to recover, balance, and purify the cholesterol overdose. What we've seen in the research is that women will manufacture a higher level of estrogen, for instance, than the other female hormones, leading to a higher estrogen load, which correlates with a higher rate of breast cancer. In men we see a higher load of downstream hormones leading to a higher rate of prostate cancer, for instance. So no cholesterol—no meat, no milk, and no eggs.

A lot of people think that coconut oil is a good alternative to other oils. Is it?

Actually, no. Here's why: there are no trees on the planet with a ready-made bottle of coconut oil, olive oil, or sesame oil for you to walk up to and pluck. So are they man-made substances or God-made substances?

Oils that exist naturally in whole foods are fine because their chemistry is completely different when we ingest them with fiber and other nutrients. When we ingest coconut meat, we can scrape off the inner part of the coconut with no difficulty. But no matter how it's extracted it's an extract, and extracts do not naturally occur in nature.

How do you recommend people dress their salads?

In *The Starch Solution*, coauthor Mary McDougall offers some wonderful salad dressings. There's a creamy, tangy, sweet, and delicious one you can make with cashews and then add garlic and lemon. It is one of my favorites.

You can also make plant-based salad dressings with no oils, which are absolutely delicious and healthy. When I'm in a restaurant, I just ask for lemons and balsamic vinaigrette, which is great.

What do you think is the biggest mistake people make when they go about healing on their own?

A major problem for many of us is that we try to resolve our concerns on our own. Einstein explained that for us to really resolve our issues, we have to think about our patterns—how we actually approach problems. He drew a small circle and suggested that what we normally do when we have a problem is see if we already know how to solve it. So we go to what we already know. He made the circle very small to indicate that what we already know is inherently very limited. Then he drew a bigger circle around the small circle and said that if we don't already know how to resolve the issue, we access information that we hope can help us do that. While going into a bigger area of what we think we need to know, we tell ourselves, "Oh, I'll just google this or I'll find it on YouTube." But not everything is on Google or YouTube.

Einstein also shared that true breakthroughs in our lives happen outside of those two circles, in what he referred to as the arena of the imagination. Imagination, he suggested, is far more important than knowledge since knowledge is inherently limited to what we know and understand while imagination embraces the entire world and all there will ever be to know and understand. Imagination is the preview of life's coming attractions. And the most effective way to tap in to imagination, as well as innovation, creativity, and insight, is through collaboration. That's what Angela did. Although brilliant, with a 4.0 grade average in high school and a challenging major in college, she finally realized, "I do not have this figured out. I need help." The first step in resolving our concerns is finding the humility to realize that we need help and then seeking help from someone who can see our blind spots. We all have them.

Once we understand and align with our divine design, we can recognize that this is how the human body was designed to work. Then we begin operating with integrity. And when that happens, we heal, we thrive, and we're happy.

WISDOM TO REMEMBER

At one moment Angela thought she was going to die from diabetes, and the next she found a doorway to life again. When one door closes for you, see if you can find another that opens. Coach Ruben is suggesting that to reverse diabetes and other life-depleting conditions, it is best to attune to your original divine design by choosing life-promoting thoughts, words, actions, friends, environments, and foods. I like to remind myself that we are made mostly of water, so it is best to eat food as closely resembling that source as possible. Water, H_2O, is made up of hydrogen and oxygen. Oxygen (O) comes from the air we breathe, while the greatest source of hydrogen (H) is the sun. Thus foods consumed closest in time to when they were exposed to the sun have the most hydrogen. Processing foods, on the other hand, dehydrates them.

When resolving concerns, using your imagination will expand your possibilities. In addition, collaborating with others, especially a mentor or mastermind, will help you see past your blind spots and get new ideas.

WHAT YOU CAN DO

To go from surviving to thriving, explore the following dietary and lifestyle recommendations:

- Focus on positive thoughts.

- Speak supportive words.

- Keep promises to yourself.

- Wisely choose the company you keep.

- Pick foods that match your divine design.

  - ~ Foods to avoid that can cause inflammation

    - ○ Dairy

    - ○ Meat

    - ○ Eggs

    - ○ Processed oils

  - ~ Foods and substances to avoid that can be toxic

    - ○ Sugar

    - ○ Fried items

    - ○ Soda

    - ○ Legal drugs like nicotine

    - ○ Caffeine

    - ○ Excitotoxins, like MSG, BHT, and aspartame

~ Foods to eat that can be energizing

- o Whole grains

- o Legumes

- o Starchy vegetables

~ Foods to eat that can enhance performance

- o All vegetables, especially leafy greens

- o Fruits

~ Healthy sources of fat

- o Nuts, seeds, and avocados (ill-advised for those with too much fat in their bodies)

~ Healthy alternatives to salad dressings made with processed oils

- o Plant-based salad dressings

  - o At home you can make a dressing with cashews, garlic, and lemon

  - o In a restaurant, order fresh lemon and balsamic vinaigrette

CHAPTER 3

Was It Love or Was It Kale?
GOODBYE LUPUS

With

BROOKE GOLDNER, MD

"Be sure you put your feet in the right place, then stand firm."

—Abraham Lincoln

Brooke Goldner, MD, best-selling author of *Goodbye Lupus* and creator of the Hyper-Nourishing Healing Protocol for Lupus Recovery, is the founder of GoodbyeLupus.com and the Smoothie Shred Community, and has been featured in multiple documentaries, media interviews, and stage appearances. I was first fascinated by her story when I heard it from her husband, who is one of my business and financial development trainers, and was even more taken by it when I later heard her tell it.

Dr. Brooke Goldner, would you tell the story of how you began having health issues in childhood and what healed you.

My story began when I was sixteen years old. I was a normal, nerdy kid enjoying my little group of friends, but weird things started to happen. I began having arthritis in different parts of my body, which is not typical of kids that age, and I couldn't figure out why. I had a passing thought maybe it was from playing volleyball, but then I reminded myself that I mostly sat bench for volleyball, so that wasn't a good explanation. At the same time, I started getting rashes, including a butterfly rash all across my face, which is typical of lupus. My energy levels plummeted. I began getting migraines that would last for days, and I would vomit from the pain. Once, after being at a pool all day with a friend, I had a migraine, vomited, and ended up with a bright red rash on my face. My dad looked at me and said, "You know, I think the skin is a window to your health. So I think we should go to the doctor." I didn't take that suggestion very seriously because my dad always jokingly spouted off what I call "dad science." But I now teach that as a truth, and something was terribly wrong.

At the hospital, I was diagnosed with lupus, a serious autoimmune disease that can spread throughout the body, affecting the heart, lungs, kidneys, and brain. My blood tests and kidney biopsy confirmed that I had stage 4 kidney failure. Because of the severity of the disease, my doctors had little hope that the medicines normally used would save my kidneys. They said if they didn't do something very radical, I might not make it past six months. The best we could hope for was dialysis, and worst-case scenario was that I would not survive.

I had a hard time taking in what was happening. I was only sixteen, and more worried about the cute guy in my biology class than life and death issues. For my family, it was devastating—I'm an only child, and my mom comes from a family of Holocaust survivors, so they had high hopes that I would do many great things.

In a desperate attempt to shut off my immune system, I was given chemotherapy in addition to high-dose steroids, which was an experimental treatment at the time. I had chemotherapy once a month for two years, from age sixteen to eighteen. It was pretty rough, but my family always kept me focused on my purpose in life and the fact that lupus was just something I was dealing with. I now give that same message to people struggling with disease, telling them: "Don't take the disease on as who you are because then everything else crumbles away and you just suffer. Instead, focus on why you're on the earth. We're not on the earth to suffer but because we have a gift we were born to give."

After each chemotherapy treatment, at least a week would pass before I could do anything except read ahead in my textbooks, which helped me stop focusing on what was happening to my body. I went from nerd to über-nerd, because I knew every answer in class. Ultimately I graduated in the top ten of my high school class and received a scholarship to my first-choice college: Carnegie Mellon University.

My last chemotherapy treatment was exactly one week before starting college, and by then the lupus had gone into remission, which was like a rebirth. Still, even in remission I had to be careful to avoid sunlight, get enough sleep, and avoid stress or I would get achy joints, migraines, or a rash. I was very careful; did really well in college; and stayed in remission those four years. My blood tests still showed that I was positive for everything in lupus, however, my kidneys were stable.

While in college, I became interested in genetic research, thinking that maybe as a genetic researcher I could help people with lupus. But I found lab work to be largely unfulfilling and realized I wanted to help people hands on. So I decided to go to medical school. My goal in life wasn't so much to cure diseases as to help people deal with suffering. I believed that you could be sick and not suffer, still be happy, and enjoy good quality of life.

The challenge with medical school was that students with an illness or disability were expected to work the same hours as everyone else. At one point I was working a hundred hours a week and my body couldn't handle it. I got sick again; ended up having a transient ischemic attack, also known as a ministroke; and passed out in one of the clinics. I was told there was no permanent damage to my brain but I was at extreme risk for a major stroke.

After the ministroke, I had to give myself injections of blood thinners in my stomach every day, supposedly for life. I was heartbroken, because having been in remission throughout college I had thought the worst was over. The ministroke instead reminded me that the clock was ticking. With lupus, people don't live long lives. The disease is constantly progressing; even medications that slow the progression can't stop it. Without the medicines

I was going to have a stroke and with them I might have a bleed—caused by a car accident, for instance—that could take me out. This new prognosis seemed like the final nail in the coffin in terms of having children since people with lupus often die in pregnancy or childbirth, due to blood clots. After a couple of weeks of mourning, I went back to thinking: *You know, I'm still here. So I'm going to finish medical school and live my dream. After all, there are people who live a long, healthy life but never live their dream.* I was once again filled with gratitude for my life.

I finished medical school and got my first-choice residency at Harbor UCLA, hoping to treat the homeless. I wanted to work with the sickest people no one else wanted to work with. However much time I had on this planet, I wanted it to be meaningful and dedicated to helping others live better and happier lives.

I was just finishing up my last rotation in medical school when I met weight-loss expert and master trainer Thomas Tadlock, the most incredible human I'd ever encountered—gorgeous and also funny, caring, and brilliant. I didn't believe in soulmates until I met him.

We fell in love fast, and within a month he was talking marriage, which was awesome, but then I had to bring up my illness. I had to tell him I wasn't going to live to a very old age, I could never have children, and he was going to end up taking care of me before I die, as I would become handicapped from joint problems and other disabilities. He paused for a moment then said, "I'd rather have a short life with you than a lifetime with anybody else." I replied, "Okay, let's get married!" I was thrilled since I'd often imagined wearing a white coat but had never let myself dream of a white dress.

Unbelievably, I healed my lupus because of vanity! I wanted to look amazing for my wedding, but, unlike everyone else I knew who had lost weight for their weddings by starving themselves, I didn't want to hurt my body. So I decided to do Thomas's nutrition program. At the time, he was working with MTV stars, young people partying too much who would then need a six-pack for their music video in three weeks. He'd train them and within three weeks they'd look smoking hot. He knew how to raise metabolism by feeding the body right.

His nutrition program for rapid fat loss included tons of raw vegetables, tons of water, and omega-3 fatty acids, but also meat. "I'm not doing the meat," I explained, having been a vegetarian since childhood. Animals were my friends, and I didn't want to eat them, though I ate a lot of eggs and dairy products, especially cheese, unaware that these products caused animal suffering as well.

So he made the program vegetarian for me, which he'd never done before. And since dairy products make people fatter, I had to give up my cheese addiction. I ended up accidentally on a hyper-nourishing 100 percent plant-based vegan diet consisting of only whole plant foods and tons of raw vegetables.

Just under four months later when we were getting ready to go to our wedding, I had blood tests that came back negative for lupus, which was medically impossible according to Western medicine. Now I know it is medically possible, because I've done it, and so have my patients. I've reversed all kinds of autoimmune diseases for people whose doctors said they couldn't be healed. My own blood tests have been negative for lupus these past thirteen years.

Looking back, it's clear that my first negative results were due to the nutrition program I had implemented, as it was the only change I had made. Previously I'd had no idea that nutrition could have any impact on lupus or most other diseases. I had actually not learned much about nutrition at all in medical school.

After four years of being very healthy, I decided to have children. I enjoyed a healthy first pregnancy and delivery, though I had to have a cesarean section because our son was in breech position, a risky procedure for someone with lupus. Afterward, the doctors were waiting around the bed as if waiting for something to happen, and I just got up and said, "When's lunch?" They were astonished. My doctors were convinced that the lupus would come back after I gave birth, but it didn't. I was healthy; our son was healthy; and I not only healed rapidly from my C-section but I was back in my pre-pregnancy jeans only nine days after giving birth.

This was when my husband and I realized that something truly remarkable had happened to my body. I was vibrant and strong; a far cry from the sickly women I had been most of my life. We realized that I wasn't only healthy but my body was responding in real time to every challenge with which it was presented.

Thomas's research had long been in nutritional and exercise science, and mine was in disease. Our combined efforts had accidentally given rise to the most low-inflammation healing diet physically possible. The superfast metabolism it generated had allowed me to rapidly lose my pregnancy weight without trying, while feeling strong and energized and producing an abundant milk supply for our child. The diet had also allowed my body to heal from autoimmune disease after being sick for twelve years. We had been given the extraordinary gift of healing, and we felt we had to share it with the world.

Before long, we started doing studies with people, the results of which were 100 percent positive. Every person who adopted our diet got increasingly healthier, so we expanded our practice.

At the time, I was the medical director at a nonprofit in Long Beach, California. Then after giving birth to our second son, I retired. Our plan was to devote ourselves full time to teaching healing and sharing our knowledge with the world.

I relate to this idea of getting a disease and then thinking that your purpose is to help people heal that disease. Initially when I got my diagnosis, that was what I thought. But then I came back to reality and decided, *Maybe I should know more about this or heal myself first.*

Beautiful. So you wanted to help people heal before you even healed. When it comes to healing yourself, it's a lot of work, so you have to have a big reason for it. For some folks, it's being a mom, or being a husband or wife. I wanted to figure out how to fix this so I could help heal the world. When you have a mission like that, it's hard for anyone to stop you.

Yes. Brooke, a lot of people try a vegan diet and give up. Would you walk us through the key aspects of a vegan diet that make this new eating pattern both sustainable and helpful in healing?

One of the biggest problems with diet and nutrition advice today is the focus on what to avoid. So when people go on diets, they feel like they're being deprived. They come to me and complain, "Well, they just eliminated my whole diet."

People are getting sicker and sicker at younger ages, and yet nobody seems to understand why. To me the reason is very clear. Most people in our country are eating a diet of all inflammatory foods and zero healing foods like vegetables, so of course they're sick. Sadly, the most commonly eaten vegetable in our country is ketchup, followed by French fries. In school lunches, ketchup counts as a serving of vegetables, which is why many kids today have plagues in their arteries by age eight. Instead, it is most healthy to have the majority of our diet come from plants. That's what our bodies are designed to use, and that's what works for healing. When people aren't ready to embrace a healing diet, telling me, "Oh my God, I'm never going to have a piece of fish again" or "I'm never going to have a piece of meat again," I tell them, "If you want to eat those foods for now, okay, but add vegetables." Over time we replace more inflammatory foods with healing plant foods, and when people feel better they get more motivated to keep going.

One way to start making your diet more healthy is to add something living to each meal. For example, if you normally eat a burger and French fries, get a burger and salad or a burger, French fries, and a salad. Then add something raw as a snack, like some broccoli and guacamole; in raw foods the nutrients are intact.

The best and easiest way that Thomas and I have found to get people to add what they're missing is by having them drink green smoothies. We created the Smoothie Shred Community to help people all over the world start embracing better health and fitness. It's focused on people adding nutrients so they can get fitter and healthier. A lot of these people are becoming vegan because they realize, "Wow, when I drink this stuff I feel like a million bucks, and then I have a burger and feel like a nap." When you start to know what your body is supposed to feel like, it's easy to give up meat, cheese, and other inflammatory foods.

In effect, we teach people how to make green smoothies that are healing. They're 75 percent greens, because greens are the most nutrient-dense foods on the planet. We put in kale or spinach, add whatever fruit makes it taste good, then add omega-3s from flax or chia seeds, and finally water, or unsweetened almond milk. These smoothies taste great. Making plants the largest portion of what you consume every day is the place to start, and then the rest of the changes become easier. If you're drinking sixty-four ounces of green smoothies a day, you don't have enough of an appetite to eat other stuff and, because you feel so good, you don't crave those foods. People post every day that their sugar cravings are going away because they're nourished, feel energized, and high just on natural energy and life.

We also advise people to make sure they are superhydrated. Most people are severely dehydrated, so we recommend at least ninety-six ounces of water a day for those trying to improve their health.

Unfortunately, it is possible to be vegan yet not healthy since so many unhealthy vegan products are sold, such as the fake meats and cheeses made out of oil. We sometimes eat those ingredients when we go out, but the majority of what goes into our bodies is food that grows on the planet, that is alive.

Would you end with a thought about the difference between healing and eliminating symptoms?

There's an important difference between what doctors normally do and what I have the honor and pleasure of doing. As a physician, I was trained to figure out how to eliminate symptoms. For example, if the blood pressure goes up, you say, "Oh, high blood pressure's not good, so let me use a medication to bring the blood pressure back down." Then when the number looks normal again, we get a false sense of security. The problem is all you did by adding medicine was cut the Check Engine light. If a Check Engine light comes on in a car, we don't think, *How do I turn off that light?* We ask, "What's wrong with the engine?" Then we go to a mechanic to fix the engine. What we do with medications is often cut off that light. But rising blood pressure is the body's way of saying, "Excuse me, there's a problem with the engine. Fix something."

Just lowering the blood pressure does not improve the health of the heart. When we see the blood pressure is up, we need to instead look at what the individual is eating that may be causing arteries to harden so the heart is working harder to push the blood through, then change the diet to get plaques to melt away and get the heart working more efficiently. The same approach is used with diabetes, when a doctor says, "Oh, there's high blood sugar. Add medicine. Look, sugar's normal again. You should be fine." What about what's *causing* the sugar to go up? People with type 2 diabetes who take their medications can still end up with shortened life spans and tragically reduced quality of life from losing their feet or their eyesight. Medicine doesn't remedy the cause of the disease, which is the consumption of animal fat, leading to insulin resistance.

When we just treat symptoms, as typically occurs in Western medicine, we get a false sense of security that we're doing something but people continue to get sicker. Many doctors get burned out because they go into medicine wanting to heal people and end up experiencing a revolving-door scenario in which people keep coming back with more and more medical problems.

By contrast, doctors who learn from me seem happier and get far better results because they're taking people off medication. Doctors do want to heal people; they just don't have all the information they need to do so. I'm a Western medical doctor, so I still prescribe medication, but I use it as a tool to keep people alive so that I can then heal them using nutrition. For instance, if someone's kidneys are failing or they're about to die of a heart attack, medications can give us time. But it's not helpful to make them the endgame, because they don't address the underlying problems.

One of the best comments I've heard recently, from a movie I'm in called *Eating You Alive*, is: "People aren't living longer, they're dying longer." Medicines treat symptoms to keep people living longer, but they're feeling like hell.

Fortunately, a medical revolution is beginning. Doctors from all over the world are learning how to treat more than symptoms through nutrition, but change is slow. People who are sick now and using nutrition to heal themselves should share their results with doctors so they can see the changes firsthand. A cardiologist I know learned from a patient who should have died but reversed her heart disease using a plant-based diet. That doctor now has a podcast teaching people plant-based nutrition and puts all her patients on plant-based diets. She told me that she is saving many more lives she never could have saved before. Her patient not only healed herself but, by sharing her healing with her doctor, she has saved many more lives as well.

We can't split the body into parts and say, "Here's your headache medicine. Here's your leg medicine. Here's your heart medicine." We need to look at the body holistically and say, "The body's giving us signals—the Check Engine lights are coming on. There's something wrong with the entire system. We need to get to the root cause of it and start reducing inflammation." Then all the other symptoms may go away and we won't need medications anymore.

Yes, doctors are starting to embrace such integrative ideas. One of my clients was supposed to get surgery for fibroids. Her doctors told her to go on a plant-based diet. Within her first week of working with me, the doctors postponed her surgery for two months. Then a week before the surgery was scheduled they looked at her lab work and told her she didn't need surgery.

Fabulous. Fibroids go away pretty quickly with a plant-based diet. Such stories give me much hope that things are getting better. Not fast enough, however. Writing this book is a great service because people need the hope it inspires. I always tell my patients, "When you heal, make a video. Let people know that others have healed this way." We need to get the word out through videos, books, and blogs so more people can hear the message and heal.

Yes. This book introduces multiple stories of healing, and others are reported through my website. The more of these stories people read, the more believable they become.

We have an extraordinary ability to heal, and we are born to heal. I always tell people that when you get a paper cut you don't have to pull out your sewing kit because your body knows what to do. It's true on the inside, too. If your thyroid gets inflamed, if you get fibroids, if you get an autoimmune disease, your body can fix it. But to do so it needs to have the right nutrients. Such healing is extraordinary to witness. With some people who have been sick for ten years, I've at first been skeptical about their potential for healing, thinking, *Gosh, I don't know. This is really severe.* But then they rapidly become symptom free and I am amazed.

One of my patients with severe lupus, scleroderma, and Sjögren's syndrome was in the ICU for four months before finding me. The doctor said he wasn't going to make it, but he's now living medication free and healthy. It is unbelievable how resilient our bodies can be when we take care of them.

Our bodies are keeping us alive right now, hoping that we're going to do something to make ourselves healthy. I'm in tears every day witnessing what can happen when people simply learn how to nourish themselves properly.

WISDOM TO REMEMBER

Following Brooke's wedding with her soul mate, her long ordeal with lupus ended. Was it love or was it kale? The only change she had made was her diet. And that new diet has helped every other person she has given it to.

If you have been diagnosed with a disease, be careful not to identify with it; instead, focus on your purpose in life. Rather than just treating symptoms, find ways to heal yourself. And remember that physical beauty comes from inner health not just of the body but also of the mind and spirit.

WHAT YOU CAN DO

It is amazing to see how people can be very sick for many years then change their diets and their diseases vanish.

When choosing foods for a healthy new diet:

- Don't worry about giving up what you love; just add more nutrient-rich foods to your diet.

- Eat living food. Make sure that 75 percent of your diet consists of vegetables or other raw foods.

- Drink at least ninety-six ounces of water a day.

- To get lots of nutrients from raw vegetables, drink green smoothies. To make a green smoothie:

  ~ Fill 75 percent of the blender with dark leafy greens, like kale or spinach.

  ~ Add whatever fruit you like, for taste.

  ~ Add omega-3 flax or chia seeds.

  ~ Add water or unsweetened almond milk to desired consistency.

CHAPTER 4

The Right Kind of Fuel
CHANGING THE DIET FOR WELLNESS

With
TARA GESLING

"Transformation literally means going beyond your form."

—Wayne Dyer

Tara Gesling is a motivational speaker, functional health practitioner, integrated nutrition health coach, organic gardening and food expert, and author of the best-selling book *The 180° Wellness REvolution: Simple Steps to Prevent and Reverse Illness*. Also the founder of Cultivating Health, LLC. She lives on a farm in central Virginia with her husband, daughter, and four dogs. When I heard the condition her body started in, I was amazed at what she has accomplished.

Tara, you have an interesting story about how you ended up healing your body beyond what anyone expected. Would you please share it.

While growing up, my family didn't like to cook very much, so we often ate TV dinners, fast food, and processed food—what today we would call the typical American diet. As a result, the nutrition I was getting was very poor. I started dabbling in gardening when I was twelve or thirteen years old. I had neighbors who had gardened and farmed their entire lives and I learned from them as much as I could. Food from my garden tasted so good! As I got older and graduated from high school, I lived in the city for a while where I didn't have access to a garden, so I relied mostly on fast food again. During annual checkups, my doctors would tell me such things as, "Your cholesterol is really high" or "Your blood pressure is really high and you're only twenty-two." Then they would say, "But you're young—don't worry about it." I didn't want to worry about it, so I didn't. Over the next few years I got flu shots as recommended and had dental work done. My dentist talked me into replacing the old silver amalgam fillings with new amalgam fillings that he claimed would be longer lasting. The procedure sounded good but led to sickness. I had no clue that there was mercury in amalgams.

Soon afterward, I started getting colds a lot. Next thing I knew, I had an accident and tore ligaments and tendons in my leg, which then wouldn't heal. I was given a tetanus shot while at the hospital, not realizing that it also contained mercury. I was the perfect patient and did everything the doctors said, yet my leg was swelling and would not get better. The condition eventually evolved into a neuromuscular disease called reflex sympathetic dystrophy (RSD). It took doctors about two years to diagnose it, and by that point I was in a wheelchair. I spent many years in a wheelchair in severe pain. The event that turned things around for me was what some people would call a near-death experience. After this experience I knew that I could get better, which started me on the road to recovery.

One of the first things I knew I had to do was stop poisoning my body. At the time, I was on about thirteen prescription medications. I had never thought to ask, "Can these drugs harm me? Have these medications been tested together for safety? Do you have any idea what they are doing to my body?" Also, when I was very ill and confused all I could do was eat fast food, frozen food, cook canned goods, maybe fry eggs—most weren't very nutritious.

As the saying goes, "When the student is ready the teacher will appear." My first teacher was a couple of years older than me and been wanting to study nutrition at the Institute for Integrative Nutrition, where I later studied. She wasn't able to travel to New York for the classes at that time, yet she still knew way more than I did! She showed me how to cook some dishes and how to keep foods on hand that I could quickly use on days when I could not function at all from the wheelchair.

During that time, I was diagnosed as having hypoglycemia, hypothyroid, Hashimoto's, rheumatoid arthritis, fibromyalgia, chronic fatigue, high cholesterol, high blood pressure, stage 3 adrenal exhaustion, irritable bowel syndrome (IBS), and more. Instead of worrying about all these labeled diseases, I was relieved when I could work on my whole body in a functional way, after which everything would start responding. I began with food; this turned out to be rewarding because within six months some feeling began to return in my injured leg, which had been numb for years.

Then I looked at emotional events in my past. I had undergone difficult experiences as a child that I had not dealt with over the years. I also explored stressors in my everyday life and became aware of internal stressors, such as what was going on with my adrenals, kidneys and liver, and my inability to detox the heavy metal poisoning.

I didn't get into this situation overnight, so naturally it took many years to turn my health around. I'm still working daily on detoxing and strengthening my organs and body.

Are you on any medication now?

No.

How does your body feel?

Pretty good. I'm very good at pacing myself and paying attention to the signals my body gives me. Occasionally I have to really slow it down, especially after pushing myself. I had a major exposure to mold five years ago, which sent me reeling backwards. But thankfully I was aware of what was happening and knew how to help myself. Working with the body functionally, the way I do with myself and clients, yields beneficial results time and time again.

Our bodies are made of energy, and energy is constantly in motion, so we will constantly change and need to adapt to new situations. Once we have the tools to understand that and to recalibrate our bodies, it seems we can heal more quickly.

Definitely. One of the coolest things I learned during my near-death experience was that I'm not defined by this body; I am a soul. I call my body my earth suit because I left it for a while and I was still me. I felt so light yet still conscious of my thoughts. When I came back into my body, it felt like I was being sucked in by a vacuum cleaner and I felt very heavy. Now I'm so aware of the energy in my body that I can tell when I have a block somewhere. And because I came back into my body with new awareness, I began doing energy work on myself. I also sought out practitioners of traditional Chinese medicine, who were vital in helping me understand my constitution. When my body tells me something, I listen.

How do emotions relate to our eating habits? And what can we do about that?

We often reach for food as a response to an emotion we feel. My personal experience was that I didn't want to deal with terrible things that happened to me as a child. I was seventy pounds overweight for many years. When I was bored or in pain, I used food to make myself feel good. Our parents frequently reward us with food, and so we think, "I'm not feeling good. I'm going to have a bowl of ice cream." We don't realize we're sabotaging ourselves when we do that. Instead of heading for the freezer, I focus on the underlying reason for wanting the ice cream, asking, "Why do I want this food?"

I don't advise deprivation; rather, I teach people how to enjoy food in a healthy way, which means not using it as a substitute for expressing buried emotions.

Let's say someone in emotional distress goes to the freezer to grab a tub of ice cream, becomes aware of why they want the ice cream and says, "I'm doing this because I want to satisfy myself emotionally," then wonders how they might make a choice that is better for their body, emotions, and spirit. What would you advise them to do?

In such a situation, one of the first questions I ask myself is, "What exactly am I craving?" Next I say, "I'm craving something that feels good." Then I ask myself, "What is it about such and such a food that makes me feel good? Am I really hungry for that right now or do I actually want something else?" Then I start writing. You would be amazed at what comes out when you keep asking yourself such questions.

Some people may have to ask themselves more questions, like, "I want this, but if I eat it then what? I will feel full and my blood sugar will go way up, then it will crash." They would write down what happens until they get to the real basis for the craving and are no longer hungry. The important thing is to have the awareness to stop yourself when your body does not really need the food and look for the reason for your hunger.

I had one client who had been overeating her entire life. We changed her habits within three weeks, and she was still maintaining her new approach five months later. Now she says, "I don't eat unless it's mealtime. I don't eat to take care of myself emotionally anymore." We really can change our habits to help ourselves heal.

I went through such a shift as well. I wasn't eating for emotional reasons, but I had food allergies and had to change my diet or not feel well. I had to give up many foods that I loved, but I quickly learned to love other foods. It can seem hard at first, but when we start taking the necessary steps we open up to a beautiful new world and don't miss the old world.

Yes. I don't miss my old world at all. It feels good when we start dealing with some of our unacknowledged emotions. In doing that, we learn a great deal about ourselves, and then we get lighter and life gets easier. It feels uncomfortable and scary at first, but if you get a good coach who can guide you, it becomes much easier.

It's also a great time to try different things. For example, during my recovery I tried different foods, especially Indian and Chinese. During what I call the "wheelchair days" which was in the early to mid-1990's, I had begun having reactions to almost everything I ate. At one point I could only eat maybe a dozen foods. I got through it by researching and learning how to heal what is now termed as dysbiosis or leaky gut. This was so important because approximately 80 percent of our immune system is in the gut. The gut also has everything to do with our neurological function and mood. We have the microbiome in our gut as well, and when they're not functioning correctly everything goes out of balance. In order to heal my body, I had to begin with the gut.

What can people do to ensure that their gut is not going to get out of balance and is going to detox the body and digest the food going through it?

I tell people to create a healthy environment in which the good organisms do not just survive but thrive. To create such an environment, you would eat organically grown foods from healthy soils, which have not been genetically modified and therefore do not contain harmful chemicals. In the United States, unfortunately, most people eat genetically modified foods containing a lot of chemicals.

How do you tell if foods are safe?

You have to learn about the sources of your foods, the companies producing them, and the distributors selling them. It's important to find out how the foods are grown and whether chemicals are used in the process—that is, whether it's organic, beyond organic, biodynamic or commercially farmed with chemicals. It's best to purchase your food from a local farmer or CSA (Community Supported Agriculture) so you can ask if they are farming with chemicals and find out how they are building and maintaining their soils. Farmers who understand the importance of healthy soil and microbes for healthy food, will be happy to answer your questions.

These days people have discovered creative ways to grow some of their foods. I've heard of neighborhoods where residents pick a yard or two to communally grow vegetables and fruits and share them. People living in a city can grow plants in pots or even in glass containers with water.

Yes. I'm certified in permaculture and am a master gardener instructor. I teach people how to grow things in really small spaces or on large farms. People can grow their own baby lettuce on a balcony in thirty days from the time they plant the seeds.

It's fascinating that you also grew up studying auto mechanics and relate maintenance of the body to that of a car. Would you tell us your thoughts about that?

We have to put the right fuel in our cars. We have to keep oil in them and make sure it doesn't get dirty to prevent problems within that system. I always ask people what they would do if a mechanic said to them, "You have a problem with your car's oil system. Instead of figuring out why this problem exists, we're going to have you put one of these pills in the oil every day so the engine won't blow up, which will cost you about fifty dollars a month." Would they put the pills in their car every day? I would say, "You've got to be kidding me, no way," because when I take my car to a mechanic I expect that mechanic to find the root cause of the problem and fix it. Yet, when we go to the doctor's office and the doctor does some tests and says, "You've got high blood pressure. Take these pills every day," most people do it without having asked the doctor to find the root cause of the problem. I want people to start thinking, *My body didn't do this before—what's going on that's causing the high blood pressure?* for example, and insist on learning the underlying causes of the condition so they can change it.

You reminded me that one of my doctors used to call me a Porsche, a type of car that needs a better grade of oil than the regular type. But I think all our bodies really need that. Imagine everyone being like a Porsche all the time—running well, fast, and with endurance because we fill ourselves with the best fuel possible.

If you put the wrong fuel in your car, it will not be running for long. Yet people put fast food, junk food, and synthetic chemicals into their bodies and expect their bodies to run like a Porsche. It doesn't work that way. People need to use the best fuel possible for their bodies to maintain optimal health.

WISDOM TO REMEMBER

Tara Gesling realized her body was filled with a low-grade contaminated fuel—from fast food to vaccines, mold, and mercury—causing numerous health challenges. She recognized that doctors hoped to clarify and remedy her condition by labeling and treating the symptoms but not the root causes of her health problems. She began healing when she started eating natural organically grown food. Then during a near-death experience, when she saw her soul as separate from her body, she gained awareness that helped her follow her instincts to get off of all medicines so she would eventually walk again. She stresses the importance of nutrition and eating organically grown foods, which have not been genetically modified, to make sure the body has the best fuel possible. To gain additional control over diet, she advises finding out the emotional causes of overeating or eating unhealthy foods.

WHAT YOU CAN DO

To make better food choices, recognize that old eating habits often satisfy emotional needs that must first be faced and addressed.

To uncover your true desires when reaching for food that is not healthy or for more than your body needs, ask yourself:

- "Why do I want this food?"

    ~ If the answer is, "I want to satisfy myself emotionally," then ask yourself the following questions and record on paper what it is that you really want.

        o "How do I take care of myself right now by making a choice that is better for my body, my emotions, and my spirit?"

        o "What exactly am I craving?"

        o "What is it about this food that makes me feel good?"

    ~ If your answer is that you really want this food, then ask yourself:

        o "If I eat it, what will happen?"

        o "Then what?"

You don't need a garden to grow your own organic food. Lettuce, for example, is incredibly easy to grow indoors. It requires minimal care, soil with microbial life, a little water, and a lot of sun light.

You will need:

Lettuce seeds, organic loose leaf and baby varieties

Medium-size container

A tray or saucer to place underneath for drainage

Clean gravel to layer under soil

Fresh organic composted soil

Directions:

- Fill container with 1" of gravel and then composted soil up to 1 inch from the top

- Sprinkle seeds on the soil.

- Add another ¼ inch of soil

- Spritz the seeds with water so soil is moist but not soaked.

- Mist the soil every morning until the seeds germinate.

- Water lightly every other day to keep the soil moist but not drenched.

- Place seedlings in the sunniest window on the south side of your house so they get 14–16 hours of sunlight per day.

CHAPTER 5

Wearing Your Medicine
Herbal Remedies for Healing the Gut

With

Mary Wutz

*"You don't learn to walk by following rules.
You learn by doing, and by falling over."*

——Sir Richard Branson

Mary Wutz is an herbalist and founder of Seam Siren, which produces sustainable medicinal clothing. She has developed a broad background in several holistic modalities, including herbalism, permaculture, reflexology, Reiki, neuromuscular therapy, and the Suzuki method of playing music. These modalities have helped in her personal healing and in becoming deeply attuned to nature and nature's connections with the human body.

Mary, would you tell us about your healing journey.

I've become very grateful for my health crisis. Until it happened I had been running my own business and was stressed out. At the time of my health crisis, I was living on a sailboat with my ex-fiancé, disconnected from the world of technology for the first time. I was loving the feeling of not having a cell phone and not having utilities to pay. I was learning how to slow down, and I was practicing Reiki energy healing every day.

It was a pretty rustic adventure. We didn't even have an engine on our boat except a little outboard motor, and we were living on a very small budget, eating fish we caught for every meal. We came to a little island, and when we interacted with the fellow who owned it I ate meat for the first time in three months and drank moonshine all night. The next day I got very sick.

I felt that I had alcohol poisoning but later found out I had contracted a beef tapeworm from a hamburger. It took me eight months to fully discover the cause of my illness. After I became sick, we sailed for three months, during which time I often felt nauseated, bloated, and had no appetite. By the time we got back to South Carolina, where we lived, my hair was falling out; every time I ate something I would throw up and my stomach would become distended; and I was having panic attacks.

Worried about my condition, I went to doctors. The doctors declared, "It sounds like you have an ulcer" or "It sounds like you have———." I went to every Western doctor possible, but nobody could tell me what actually was wrong. Or they put me on anti-anxiety medication, which didn't help.

Then I experienced what I like to call a divine intervention. One day I was drawn to an office across from where I worked out and met a nurse who had been trained in many different holistic modalities. She had two dachshunds, ages eighteen and twenty-one, that drank alkaline water, and she fed them a raw diet. It was my first exposure to this way of thinking and the first time I had ever seen a far infrared sauna or an alkaline water machine.

She explained, "You've got all the symptoms of a parasitic infection." Within a week I had the appropriate testing, which confirmed the diagnosis. I had a beef tapeworm that was estimated to be three meters long by that time because I'd had it inside me for so long, as well as an Asiatic yeast infection and other problems. Once your gut lining has been compromised by a parasite, you get food allergies and a whole cascade of things happening in your GI tract. (Always very sensitive, I had tended toward those types of problems as a child. My parents called me "the high-maintenance child," but now I say I'm highly refined—something I think happens to lots of highly sensitive people.) After getting the diagnosis, I took a pharmaceutical that killed the tapeworm, and it came out in pieces. The parasite had eaten my stomach lining—the part of the body that protects us from pathogens and all sorts of contaminants that are in our food. Once you have a parasite that compromises your stomach lining, it's very easy to get other parasites because there's bacteria in all foods. As a result, I started getting wave upon wave of adverse reactions to food as I was developing food allergies to almost everything.

My father was in the pharmaceutical insurance business, so I had grown up with a strictly Western approach to illness. I got chronic sinus infections and was sick all the time as a child. Now I realize that I was sick all the time because I was fed antibiotics like candy, and was eating dairy and wheat, which contributed to my illness. Antibiotics, which are not specific enough to kill only bad bacteria in the gut, kill the good bacteria, too. In doing so they create an imbalance in proper gut flora, which can lead to depression, leaky gut, poor food assimilation, and weight gain, among more serious conditions—all of which can be helped by probiotics and digestive enzymes, which can help down food. Still reeling from the aftereffects of decades of antibiotics, I was receptive when the nurse who correctly diagnosed me with a parasite offered, "There are plants that I think would really work for you in a tea—comfrey, calendula, and meadowsweet."

She recommended using the far infrared sauna, drinking alkaline water, taking supplements like hydrochloric (HCl) to help my digestive tract fire enough to kill off some pathogens, and going on an elimination diet. Consequently, for an entire year I only ate yams, the one food to which I didn't have reactions. A Chinese medicine practitioner told me that's because the yam is a toning food, and another woman explained that root vegetables repair the gut lining. I also began drinking the tea recommended by the nurse three to five times a day, which is what ultimately repaired my leaky gut. Then I started noticing that I could add some other foods without having reactions, but it took me about two and a half years to heal. I wouldn't even say I'm fully rebalanced now. When you basically lose your topsoil—the immune lining in your stomach—it's a big deal. I'm even more sensitive now than I was before. Taking probiotics is always going to be a part of my life to avoid having symptoms.

As we consciously go down the spiritual path, part of being sensitive is having the ability to tune in to more things. But it can feel challenging because we're tuning in to all things good and bad, and we have to figure out how to process all that we've sensed and absorbed.

Exactly. After my leaky gut was repaired, I ended my relationship, moved to California, and studied herbalism at California School for Herbal Studies. I also attended Living Light Culinary Institute to study food science. There I got to know about thirty or forty plants well. In addition, I learned how we're all biochemically different and how our bodies have different reactions to various foods—how, for example, the body breaks down sesame seeds as opposed to how it breaks down sesame oil or tahini. We may have a reaction to one but not the other. A lot of people have allergies to certain foods without understanding why.

After completing school, I was mentored by medical herbalist David Hoffman. Then I started helping my friends and family. Later, when I got more confident about my abilities, people I didn't know would come to me. Following the law of attraction, these were mostly people with GI disturbances or hormone imbalances. I also began a spiritual practice.

While doing a lot of healing in connection with thought patterns and belief systems, I came to understand more about how my fear and anxiety had been exacerbated both by the parasite and because I wasn't absorbing amino acids to make the hormones that calm me. I also traveled around the world studying ancient traditions and how different tribal communities used various plants for healing. I spent lots of time in isolation with these teachers, including shamans and herbalists, absorbing everything I could about how various cultures view healing.

I discovered that approaches to healing differ widely among cultures. In Maui, where I now live, when people are sick they first look at family relationships. So if you come down with a cold they consider what family members you are not getting along with, and those family relationships are what they heal first. A lot of other cultures first heal the emotional or spiritual parts of people. Only Western cultures focus first on people's physical aspects. After learning about culturally different approaches to healing, I started incorporating that knowledge into my own practice.

Over time, my intuitive abilities became further developed. It's hard to discern energies coming through and hard for the body to relax—elements essential to healing—when you are inundated with the many different wavelengths and technologies characteristic of modern society. I always ask clients about their environments and jobs, and I take a look at how stressful their daily lives are, because a stressful lifestyle is probably the biggest hurdle for people seeking to heal. That's one reason I live in Maui now. Living a quieter, less stressful lifestyle is one of the most helpful things people can do when healing themselves, as it was for my own healing.

People experience significant shifts toward improved health when they make such changes. There are many different modalities that can support us, but healing basically depends on getting into a stress-free state, treating your body like a temple, and eating good food.

I understand the toll that stress takes on a person's health. Once I had a very stressful job and took a couple months off. People who saw me after a month or two of being away from work exclaimed, "You look at least two years younger."

Nice. Initially, I was trained by studying textbooks about body chemistry so if people are sick I could create a protocol that made sense in light of textbook discussions about such things as antimicrobials, polysaccharides for immune system support, and adaptogens for stress response. Then, while creating these protocols I started to hear little voices in my head saying things like "red clover," which didn't make sense in the cases I was involved with. I talked to my mentors and felt the plants were talking to me, saying, "Hey, I'm here to help this person. I'm the one they need."

For a long time I didn't listen to these voices, but in the last few years I've embraced the fact that one of the gifts I have is to help people find their "plant allies." Plants can help us in so many ways, for both environmental healing and personal healing. They are on the planet to co-create healing with us. Before 1908, our medicine came from plants; only after 1908 did pharmaceutical companies regularly start making synthetic drugs.

Being an herbal healer is a little like being an alchemist assessing people's personalities, situations, and other variables then looking in a toolbox of plants for medicines to heal them. For any ailment, there's usually a plant that resonates with the frequency of the person. For example, specific plants work better with sensitive people, who don't need the super powerful plants that are needed by less sensitive people. If somebody is suffering a lot, one of my favorite plants to use is calendula, which has a nurse-like energy—it's saying, "Don't worry. I will take care of you." It's like a support system.

I can imagine that different plants do affect people quite differently. When I used to take allopathic medicines prescribed by doctors, I would tell them that I was having severe headaches or this or that reaction, and they would say, "It doesn't do that." But despite what they said I still had those reactions.

A good example of how various plants affect people in different ways is valerian root. Many people take valerian root as a sedative for sleep, but it actually stimulates 15 percent of people.

During my travels, I became very interested in how medicinal clothing has been used in many cultures to promote healing by absorption of substances through the skin. For example, in India thousands of years ago if a person had an ailment that was similar to what we would now call arthritis, their clothing was dyed in turmeric. In Ayurveda there's something called *ayurvastra* or healing cloth. This is a process where they combine various medicinal plants to create healing dyes. There's also something called chromotherapy, which is the science of using colors to adjust body vibrations to frequencies that promote health and harmony.

Wearing medicinal clothing is a healing tradition that hasn't resurfaced until now. About five or six years ago, while isolated in the jungle with a specific plant I was studying I came across an article about the medicinal uses of nettle fiber. The Nepalese people use nettle fiber when they have what we would call eczema or psoriasis. A natural antihistamine, nettle is also great for people with allergies. Nettle is nutritive and safe for almost everybody, including pregnant women. It has no well-known severe herb drug interactions, and so I like to call it nature's multivitamin. Additionally, the nettle plant sequesters carbon from the atmosphere and stores it in the soil which is extremely beneficial for the environment.

I researched more about colors and frequencies to see how natural plant dyes in fabrics can help heal parasites among other ailments. Then a year ago, I launched a new clothing company with the tag line "Wear Your Medicine." It is based on the ancient knowledge that the fibers we wear can affect us because the skin is the body's largest organ. The skin also provides information about an individual's health. When anything shows up on the skin, it's a sign that something is internally off. Usually the liver is overburdened. Chemicals from the synthetic materials people wear are themselves absorbed into the bloodstream. Studies show that such absorption has affected children.

Then, too, the fashion industry uses harsh chemical compounds that affect the environment. While some clothing companies are doing good things, more often than not companies are not doing things the right way. The fashion industry is the world's second largest contributor to CO^2 emissions. And to keep up with fashion trends, people are buying so many clothes that, as I've been told, one-fifth of our landfills consists of clothing.

Are there any popular clothing companies people can trust?

I don't want to mention specific companies, but I will say that I don't trust the terms "eco-friendly," "sustainable," or "organic" because they are essentially marketing terms. Manufacturers can say their merchandise is eco-friendly, sustainable, or organic to help people feel good about buying these products, but few such labels actually mean anything. I recommend looking into the supply chain of various companies to determine the credibility of their advertising claims.

I'm passionate about transparency and being able to trace the entire production cycle. Most companies don't do that because it's too expensive, and they are more profit-driven than socially responsible. In the supply chain that I rely on, no chemicals are used and all the work is done by hand. The biggest footprint I'm making is bringing fiber from Nepal to the United States so I can do production locally in Portland and natural fiber dying in Seattle.

My line is not only supportive of personal wellness but also compostable. And it has created a new revenue stream for Nepalese people since a fungus coming over from China is destroying their lychee crops, which is how they make most of their money.

It's equally advisable to find out where and why companies are making clothing overseas; it's often not only because it's cheaper but because there is no sufficiently skilled labor force in the United States. I am currently in discussion with a garment factory about establishing a trade school in Portland to create the needed skilled labor force. We need to raise the bar in the production of garments. I hope that my practice of being transparent and responsible in garment production will influence other businesses.

WISDOM TO REMEMBER

In her journey of healing from a parasite, Mary Wutz learned that even once a parasite is gone the lining of the stomach and digestive tract may need to be repaired to heal leaky gut and prevent allergic reactions. She also gained the awareness that a stressful lifestyle is one of the biggest hurdles to healing and discovered the importance of treating the body like a temple and eating good food.

She discovered that most non-Western cultures look first at nonphysical reasons for disease and that plants were used as medicine long before synthetic drugs were made by pharmaceutical companies. She now encourages people to discover the "plant allies" that can be beneficial to their healing and to consider the potential of wearing medicinal clothing.

In her clothing business, she is acutely aware that any chemical footprint left behind is harmful to our health and the environment, Mary is a role model in transparency of production and in minimizing humankind's adverse impacts on the environment.

WHAT YOU CAN DO

- If you have taken a lot of antibiotics, probiotics and digestive enzymes are helpful in improving digestion.

- If you want some nurturing energy, use calendula.

- Nettle fiber helps with eczema, psoriasis, and other skin conditions. It is a natural antihistamine and good for people with allergies and for pregnant women. It is considered nature's multivitamin and is beneficial for the environment as well.

- To use calendula or nettle:

    ~ Drink it in a tea.

    ~ Take it in a tincture.

    ~ Use it as a flower essence.

PART III

Body Dynamics and Healing

CHAPTER 6

Do What You Can Do

PHYSICAL THERAPY FOR STROKE AND ACCIDENT PATIENTS

With

PETER LEACH

*"When something is important enough,
you do it even if the odds are not in your favor."*

—Elon Musk

Peter Leach has been in Canada's fitness industry for over thirty years as a competitive strength athlete, martial arts competitor and instructor, and a personal trainer. He works with all types and ages of clients for weight loss, muscle building, functional training, and rehabilitation from motor vehicle accidents, yet his passion is to help people who have had strokes regain a higher level of functioning. I met Peter when he facilitated the most challenging personal development process I have ever done where his role demanded more love and courage than I had ever seen.

Peter, how did you begin helping stroke patients? And would you share a story about one person you helped.

I got into helping stroke patients by accident. Four and a half years ago an old friend, Tamara, had a stroke due to a medical error. The doctors had blocked off the left side of her left carotid, which had an impact on the functioning of the right side of her body.

Rehabilitation here in Canada generally involves being in the hospital for about a year, during which time patients are taught basic moves needed to perform daily tasks. When I first saw Tamara after her hospital stay, she was a shell of the woman I had known. She couldn't walk without a cane, her wrist was seized like a claw hand, and she didn't have a lot of mobility through the right side of her body. Her face was literally gray, her eyes dead, and she seemed to have given up on life.

I decided that it was not acceptable for my friend, who was now thirty-four, to live the rest of her life like this. That's when I became a personal trainer rather than an office worker. I was able to spend six hours a week with Tamara initially. Her sister became a yoga therapist also to help her.

Since then, some talented massage therapists and chiropractors have helped advance the system I had begun developing as a personal trainer, which involves building and rebuilding muscle. I also do a lot of work rebuilding muscle and reestablishing neural connections with people who have had motor vehicle accidents.

I don't get paid for most of what I do because when people have a stroke or accident they go on a disability pension and can't afford my services. But once I meet them I can't walk away. Many of these people become suicidal because suddenly the lives they had have been taken away from them. I've done 450 hours of volunteer work, experimenting with different people and ways of doing things because everybody's different.

Would you tell us more about Tamara's recovery?

She'd had an arteriovenous malformation (AVM), a surface brain bleed, since childhood. To repair an AVM, surgeons go in through the leg femoral artery and up through the carotid. During Tamara's surgery, they pierced an artery, and when they were bringing it back through on the left side stuff leaked out so it blocked off her carotid and essentially killed the left side of her brain. She couldn't do anything by herself, but this woman, all four foot eleven of her, became one of the toughest human beings I'd ever met.

She had been a very active woman who spent a lot of her time in the gym, hiking, and playing with her two children, and in an instant that was taken all away from her. For two hours I assessed her lack of mobility. Then with determination, I declared, "I promise I will make you better."

The fun part was watching Tamara come back bit by bit. I used to call her feisty, and I could see that quality gradually return as her body started to heal and as she gained an increased capacity to understand and speak. Along with the stroke itself affecting her body, she had what's called aphasia, which affects cognitive and speaking abilities. The fact that she was very open to trying new methods and very determined played a significant role in her recovery.

What did doctors say was possible for her?

Basically nothing. They told her she'd never again be able to walk without a cane, to use her right hand, get her arm straight, walk straight, lift her arm, hike, or to do any of the things she used to do.

At the beginning, I instructed, "Make a list of the things the doctor said you could not do ever again." As she improved her mobility and other skills, we checked them off one by one, which we have continued to do.

She got her driver's license back this year. I always teased her before her health problems that I wouldn't ride in a car she was driving because she was the scariest driver on the face of the planet. But I go riding with her now, and she's much more attentive. She has a specially adapted car that is controlled on the left side.

She had a seizure due to a high fever, unfortunately, that set her back three months, but the weird thing was it allowed her to speak better.

What I've been seeing in terms of physical and emotional changes, including changes happening to the planet right now, is that often things get worse before they get better. Part of why that happens may be because as things get worse we become more aware of the issues and therefore

better able to provide the energy necessary to help shift them in the opposite direction.

Absolutely. Some of my life coaching with Tamara involved increasing her awareness about her potential and about the good resulting from her stroke. That message was tough for her to take in until I asked, "Do you realize that my team's rehabilitation program was developed because this happened to you, that you discovered a strength you didn't know you had, and that you were planning to drift through life but now are an inspiration to my other clients?"

Now she's not going to let the stroke dictate that she can't take care of her kids, make dinner, clean the house, or do laundry. Strength comes not from what you are told you can't do but from your determination to do what you can do. I can lift some ridiculously heavy weights, but, despite being half my size, she's stronger than I'll ever be because she's had to deal with something I can't even imagine.

Would you give us an example of one of the major contributing factors helping to change such patients.

We show them what they can do as opposed to what they can't do. A lot of people who have had strokes compensate by using muscles they're not supposed to use.

Too often medical practice today masks problems rather than finding where they originate and discovering solutions. We, however, look at which neural pathways are affected, from the spine down the thoracic and through the lumbar spine, to pinpoint which nerves are being blocked. A lot of the blockage happens through what is called the pec minor, which inserts into the shoulder. If you're an office worker, pull your shoulders back to avoid having them tighten up and cause arm and shoulder problems, which could happen since a lot of the innervation and blood supply flows through there to the arms.

We start loosening that area through stretching and manipulation. Then the arms loosen up because the nerve chain feeds through the shoulders. Recently we've also started working through the rear shoulders, an area that can affect people's ability to move their arms backward and control movements down through the forearm, wrist, and fingers. The big question is, how do we get that nerve pathway to start to fire again? A lot of the problem results from doing arm movements using the trapezius muscle, which is not supposed to be used. We teach clients to do the movements without using that muscle.

At the gym one day a friend of mine was using something called a voodoo band, a two-inch-thick, seven-foot-long piece of rubber that cuts off the blood supply. We would hold the muscle in place while he ran through the exercise. We tried that with Tamara, and within a week and a half her arm was hanging normally, and she had some movement through her wrist again because we released the muscle that was holding it back and restored the innervation that had been blocked. The funny thing was she didn't even notice when this change occurred because her arm had been like that for so long she had stopped paying attention to it. Now when you look at her you would not notice anything out of the ordinary. That's huge for her recovery, for her self-esteem, and for her kids.

I believe that fitness is a lifetime endeavor. It is the element that contributes more than anything else to quality of life. Fitness not only makes activities easier but greatly enhances confidence, mental clarity, stress relief, and personal power.

Where do your vision and ideas about fitness and physical rehabilitation come from?

I opened myself up to higher powers and universal energy quite a while back. I didn't know anything about stroke rehabilitation besides the anatomical knowledge I learned as a trainer. I didn't know what effect different muscle groups had on other muscle groups until I took a neurokinetic therapy course. For example, I would be working with somebody, and I'd get the thought in my head that I need to try this or that. Since I'm open, ideas are put in front of me because they're supposed to be there and because I want them to be. During sessions I'll ask whether I should do such and such, and the answers come through very clearly: yes, no, try this, or try that.

What made you start opening up more to universal energy a few years back?

I attended a couple of courses at Success Resources America and then was inspired to go to what they call Enlightened Warrior Training Camp. It's a program that helps you discover the path you are supposed to follow—your mission. Initially, working out was a hobby. When Tamara's stroke occurred, I realized I liked being a personal trainer and helping to rehabilitate others.

For thirty-seven years I lived my life very angry and unable to relate to other human beings on an emotional level, but through my experience at Enlightened Warrior Training Camp I became a different man, open to new ideas and feelings; with the realization that what I was doing was not serving me or the people around me; with the certainty that I was being pulled in a direction to do something different. After the camp, I quit my office job, a comfortable government position with a great salary and benefits, and became a personal trainer. I've never been happier.

Do you work differently with regular clients than with those who have had strokes or accidents?

I don't treat clients who have had strokes or injuries any differently than I do guys who do power-lifting because if treated as victims they can't accomplish anything. In fact, I push them in ways that I sometimes wouldn't do with ordinary clients because that's how their bodies need to be treated. I'll be gentler with people who have been hurt in accidents because I need to be, but people who have suffered strokes are tough and they'll take the pain without even flinching. If you want a definition of what tough is, come watch the clients in rehab.

What is an exercise anyone who has had a stroke can do to improve their mobility?

Although no two clients are alike, some things can provide increased muscle stimulation and strength for all clients. Muscle tapping has been used frequently to increase stimulation and help re-create the brain-muscle connection. As a limb is being moved, the therapist will firmly tap the muscle when it is contracted and extended to activate muscle fibers and nerve connection. This can also be done with the use of a Tens machine applied directly to the muscle being exercised. Through experimentation, I have also found that muscles can be exercised through the eccentric, or lengthening, movement of the muscle. Using this method to rebuild muscle over time can also lead to increased strength and mobility when done with the concentric, or shortening, movement of muscles. Tapping can be applied to this type of movement as well.

What's the best advice that you could give somebody who has suffered from a stroke or knows someone who has?

In a television interview we did with Tamara not that long ago, she capped it perfectly when she said, "Don't give up." I would advise not being resigned to what might appear to be a permanent undesirable condition. Realize that there are people who can and want to help. Be open to alternatives and possibilities. If your doctor has claimed you can't do something, this doesn't mean it's true, because doctors often don't want to take responsibility for saying their patients can get better. Realize that you *can* get better. We've proven such outcomes with clients time and time again.

Also, if your old life is no longer possible create a vision for a new life. Consider inspiring or mentoring other individuals who have had a stroke or accident. Know that, because of your experience, your story is now so powerful that you can change others' lives through your words and actions, through who you have become because you didn't give up. Be the inspiration.

WISDOM TO REMEMBER

Peter Leach envisioned new possibilities for people who had lost mobility due to a stroke or motor vehicle accident. He kept his mind open to new ways to help people restore their mobility and gain a new lease on life despite a bleak medical prognosis. After healing beyond what the doctors and therapists had predicted, Peter's friend and client Tamara advised, "Don't give up." Peter stresses how strength comes not from listening to what you are told you can't do but from believing in your potential for progress and in doing what you can do to heal.

WHAT YOU CAN DO

To increase mobility in any part of your body that is not functioning to its full capacity:

- Have a therapist or friend tap all over the muscles of the area while you bend and tense as much of it as you can.

- Use a Tens machine on the muscles being exercised.

CHAPTER 7

No False Promises

Yoga Therapy for Inside and Out

With

Nicole DeAvilla

"There is no beauty greater than the smile of peace and wisdom glowing on your face."

—Paramhansa Yogananda

Nicole DeAvilla is a best-selling author, speaker, yoga educator, and coach with over thirty-five years of experience. She was introduced to me as a well-respected yoga therapist at the Expanding Light Retreat Center, founded by Swami Kriyananda. Her latest book, *The 2 Minute Yoga Solution: FAST and EASY Stress and Back Pain Relief*, for ANYONE at ANYTIME highlights the benefits of yoga in a fast-paced modern life.

Nicole, do you have any stories about turning things around for somebody who was not expected to heal or helping someone avoid a surgical procedure?

I do. One of those stories is of a woman who had a meniscus tear in her knee. She had tried physical therapy without success, so doctors advised surgery, which she was hesitant about. I explained, "We can work with your knee issue now because even if in the end you need surgery the work we do now will help you recover faster."

So we worked together, and she got rid of her knee pain and didn't need to have surgery. I never see somebody's limitations but instead work toward their potential.

How did she feel going through that process and seeing success?

She was very happy to not have knee surgery. As a yoga therapist, I wasn't just working with her knee. She had Hashimoto's. She had other musculoskeletal issues. I focus on a person's complete medical history and what their potential is for achieving health, happiness, and their goals in life. It made her believe in yoga therapy and her own potential for healing.

What sorts of changes did she make in her life as a result of that holistic approach?

She learned to slow down. She was a businesswoman who owned multiple stores. During that time, she sold one of her stores and became a grandmother. I helped her to psychologically and emotionally let go of something that had been important to her at one time so she could make space in her life to be a grandmother and see her daughter more often.

What did you do to help her let go of one of her stores and create more space for family?

A lot of breathing techniques and affirmations in addition to the yoga therapy she did for her body. I always lead people through complete movement for their bodies while focusing on breathing and affirmations. I help people get in touch with their inner selves so they feel they are enough and don't need to have so many external possessions and activities. People don't have to be busy all the time. I helped her gain the perspective that we go through different phases of life, sometimes being active in the external world and other times being more oriented to our inner selves, when breathing and meditation practices become a priority.

Is it typical of yoga therapy to look at the whole person or is your approach unique?

Any good yoga therapist should look at the whole person. I may be more detail oriented and willing to look at lifestyle and other factors more deeply. One issue I'm known for is musculoskeletal work - bones, muscles, ligaments, tendons so a lot of my clients see me for problems such as knee, shoulder or back pain. I've done published research on knees, shoulders and breathing. More than some yoga therapists, I go beyond the original agenda if the client is ready for it, whether it's working with their lifestyle, chakras, subtle energy, emotions, spirituality or getting in touch with their life purpose. Often it's physical pain that brings people to me. Then I check in with each client to see what else I can do for their overall well-being. Some people simply want me to fix an injury and they are done. But most people who get a taste of what yoga therapy can do for them want more.

How did you get involved with yoga therapy?

I'm one of the pioneers of yoga therapy. I was introduced to yoga in college. I grew up being very active—training horses, dancing, running—and had multiple injuries from being an athlete at a very young age. After college I became less active while working at a desk job which flared up some of those injuries. As a result of all of the sitting and previous injuries, I had pain radiating down my neck, arms, legs, and upper back. I also felt I was experiencing an emotional downward spiral along with the physical pain.

Lo and behold, one of the people I worked with was, Lila, who later became Swami Kriyananda's cook. She told me about the Ananda Yoga Center. I took the Ananda Yoga Teacher Training, initially to make myself feel better. But I was blown away by the meditation and the spiritual work with energy and the chakras. I think people come to me through the doorway of physical pain because I trained in yoga due to having physical pain myself. Because of the many musculoskeletal injuries in my body and five major surgeries I underwent before the age of twenty, I was able to experiment with healing myself of many injuries and other issues. I also learned about the emotional root causes of physical pain, how we can work with energy, and how we can shift our thoughts. Having seen the benefits of these practices myself, the day after I finished yoga teacher training I started teaching yoga out of my home.

Soon I started attracting students who had injuries. I did further training in the field of yoga therapy and also learned on the job working for a chiropractor and as a research assistant at the first Center for Sports Medicine Center in San Francisco. I was one of the pioneer yoga therapists who didn't attend a formal program - because they did not exist at the time. I consulted with doctors and swamis. I also read and got a lot of firsthand knowledge through my own yoga practice and conscientiously working with students and clients with injuries, illness and those in need of stress relief.

Would you explain what chakras are.

Chakras are subtle energy centers, or plexuses, in the spine, from which energy flows out into the nervous system and then the body, sustaining and activating its different parts. In addition to each chakra's corresponding physical realm, there are emotional, mental, and spiritual aspects that relate to the psyche and spirit. Understanding how the chakra system works and how to keep it in balance is pivotal to healing.

What was the pivotal moment that led to your relief from back pain?

When I was in the Ananda Yoga Teacher Training, my teachers shared that if you look into the eyes of a saint it will help you enter into a deep state of meditation. I craved meditation, but my back hurt so much that I ended up meditating on worsening back pain. Then one day I was determined to meditate, so I thought I would try the method of looking into the eyes of a saint. However I didn't have any pictures of a saint. One of the books we were supposed to read was *The Path*, by Swami Kriyananda, which had his picture on the cover. I didn't know him well at the time, but he seemed saintly, and indeed I found out later that he is very much a saint. So I put all of my energy and will into focusing intently on his picture looking into his eyes and then trying to meditate on them. It was not easy, but I finally found myself in a deep meditative state and my back pain disappeared! After I came out of the meditation, the pain was there again but still that was a huge turning point. I found it miraculous that I had had constant back pain and, while meditating, suddenly experienced no pain. From then on I was hooked on meditation.

I've heard that one time when Swami Kriyananda was sick and could barely breathe somebody came to visit him. The people who were watching over Swami asserted, "No, you can't come in. He's sick." But the person insisted, "I had a meeting with him. I want to see him." Suddenly, Swami came downstairs in his robe not appearing to be sick. Then the person left, and Swami got back into bed barely able to breathe again.

According to another story, a concrete well once dropped on the foot of his guru, Paramhansa Yogananda, causing him great pain. He would show people that if he centered all his energy in his spiritual eye, the point between the eyebrows, the pain in his foot would disappear then return when he again focused on his foot.

I had a similar experience while using yoga techniques to stop pain. When I was a mom with young children, late one night after everybody else was in bed I was writing about one of my mentors, Reverend John Laurence, another direct disciple of Paramhansa Yogananda. I was sleep deprived and had been sitting too much. My six-year-old daughter had fallen asleep with her dad in our bed. Typically, I would mindfully pick her up and take her to her bed, but this time I did all the things I knew not to do. When picking her up, I leaned over too far from my center of gravity, and my sacroiliac joint went out, causing excruciating intense back pain. I dropped her, fortunately onto the bed, and I fell to the floor. Everybody woke up, and I said, "Just put a blanket over me. I just need to breathe. I can't move. The pain is really bad." It was hard to even breathe without causing more pain, let alone move. While lying there breathing softly with a pain relieving breath technique, I discovered, I was focused on the pain but soon realized that was not helpful. Instead, I focused intently on the happy moments before the pain, thinking of my daughter and my son and of writing about the inspirational Reverend John Laurence. Before long I entered into an ecstatic state of joyfulness, though I still had pain.

That was another pivotal moment, helping me understand that even if we can't get rid of pain we do not need to be unhappy. I was able to experience deep joy despite the pain.

It's important for people to hear that. Would you share more about how you were able to see that you could heal and help people.

By having an optimistic outlook along with being realistic, by balancing my yoga practice with reading about science and learning techniques from others; by being in touch with my intuition and energy and by knowing that we all have potential that we often don't realize. I don't promise clients that I can heal them. I tell them I do know of things we can do together that will improve their lives, help them feel better, be happier, and perhaps achieve the full healing goals they have in mind. When they ask how long it will take, I say I don't know and encourage them to just get started. I think adopting that attitude has made the difference for me in my practice, because as soon as we say we can heal people or keep them from having surgery that's the ego speaking. Then our ability to listen to our intuition disappears, and we don't really help people as well.

I think that not promising them something unattainable also helps people relax around me. And then sometimes magical things happen.

How does healing vary in different individuals, and how would you describe healing?

One good thing to do as a yoga therapist is ask people what their level of pain is on a scale of one to ten. Otherwise, people who are still in pain, even if it is reduced, can feel like the therapies aren't working. If they are at level five or six, they can feel dejected unless you remind them that when they first came in they were at level eight or nine. Then they realize they are making progress and the therapies are in fact helping.

Naturally people want no pain, whether physical or emotional, so part of the work is to educate clients about the pattern of healing. This involves telling them that healing is taking place even if they are not at zero pain and that, while they may get to zero, their path of healing may go up and down in the meantime. As long as the healing trajectory is overall upward, they don't need to worry about the low points. And because it may take a while after injuring ourselves either emotionally or physically for those areas in the body or psyche to be reactivated, people may feel pain there again until sufficient time has passed.

People often have multiple issues, so you have to work with them from the ground up. A lot of people on a spiritual path or doing yoga just want to work on the upper chakras or energy centers, after which, though they have moments of feeling good, their pain keeps recurring. You've got to get down into the first, second, and third chakras and do work there to help them. The same is true on the physical plane: for someone with problems throughout the body, you've got to start at the base first. For example, lower back pain may result from the weight of your foot being improperly placed on the floor, which then affects your knee and hip, causing your back pain.

Deep healing takes place when people work collaboratively with their yoga therapist. Some new clients tell me to make them feel better. I take them through a session, and they feel better. Then they go out and do the same things as before, or say a little affirmation or make a tiny change, and keep coming back with little progress. Only after realizing the importance of putting their own initiative and power into the healing equation do they learn to do more for themselves; otherwise, it's like me telling them to take a pill. Until they're ready to own that their physical condition is largely a result of lifestyle or inner issues, they may keep living with the same mindset and coming back. Of course, sometimes people need nurturing week after week to eventually get to a place where they're ready to make deeper changes. And that's OK. Sometimes just showing up for your yoga therapy sessions is taking the initiative that is needed.

Being an active participant in the process is indeed very helpful. A lot of people experience this with medicine. If they stop taking medicine, the symptoms come back. It's as if the underlying issue doesn't get resolved.

Sometimes a yoga therapist, or other specialist, can be like the medicine until people more actively participate in their healing.

For this reason, I am doing more coaching. Sometimes when people see me as a coach they understand that they have a responsibility too, and become more active participants in their healing.

Is there something either in *The 2 Minute Yoga Solution* or another source that people could do right away to help with their healing?

Yes. There are many routines in *The 2 Minute Yoga Solution* book that most people will be able to comfortably and successfully practice. There is a 2 Minute Yoga YouTube Channel with simple practices on it as well.

Certainly breath work can help in healing and your readers can try some deep breathing on their own right now. A lot of scientific research shows how working with the breath helps to reduce pain, reverse the stress response in your body, and helps you to be more present in the moment so you gain greater awareness of your situation.

While doing breath work, sit upright keeping the spine in its natural curves, though you can have support if you want it. Take some full deep breaths, slowly inhaling and exhaling. Close your eyes if you wish. Keep your shoulders, throat, neck, jaws, and belly relaxed. Inhale all the nurturing, love, and joy that you need and exhale any disharmony.

Bring all your attention to inhaling and exhaling. As you continue taking deep breaths, let each one be the most important one. Feel cleansed and centered in the present moment. Then when you're ready, finish on an exhalation. Lift the corners of your mouth into a smile, and open your eyes.

I call that "smileasana."

WISDOM TO REMEMBER

As a yoga therapist, Nicole DeAvilla works with the whole body, inside and out, taking her clients' life histories into account. She has seen the power that spiritual experiences can have on healing, and stresses that inner healing is most important. She makes no false promises about physical healing and believes that people can be happy and even improving when they are physically in pain. Also active participation from the client is necessary to clear the root of an issue.

WHAT YOU CAN DO

To reduce pain and the stress response in the body, and be more present, practice the following breathing exercise:

- Sit upright with a neutral spine.

- Slowly inhale and exhale deeply.

- Close your eyes, and, keeping your body as relaxed as possible, let each breath be the most important thing happening at the moment.

- Imagine you are exhaling disharmony and inhaling all the nurturing, love, and joy you need.

CHAPTER 8

What the Cavemen Had on Us

SEEING AND WALKING AGAIN

With

MEIR SCHNEIDER, PhD

"It always seems impossible until it's done."

—Nelson Mandela

Meir Schneider, PhD, LMT, healed himself of congenital blindness and developed an original holistic approach to health. A globally respected therapist and educator, he is also the author of several bestselling books, including *Vision For Life* and *Movement for Self-Healing*. His latest book, *Awakening Your Power of Self-Healing*, is published by the Self-Healing Press. During one of his workshops, a few minutes of Meir's eye exercises cured a headache that I'd had for a few days.

Meir, would you tell us about your situation as a child—how you were born blind and how you healed that condition.

I was born with cataracts, which are uncommon in children. My two children were also born with cataracts, possibly from a genetic transmission. A cataract is an opacity of the lens, which is supposed to accommodate and transfer light.

What is especially interesting about my story is that I was born to deaf parents. I had five unsuccessful cataract surgeries. They cut my eye lens into small pieces, resulting in 99 percent of it becoming scar tissue. Most people start to develop their vision at age eight weeks and complete it at two and a half, but I missed all that development time and read Braille until I was nearly seventeen, when I learned eye exercises that helped restore my vision. Despite still having a major difficulty in my lens, these days I can read, write, and drive.

Would you share more about those exercises and how they changed your eyesight?

The exercises are based on nine principles, which today are difficult to practice naturally. Among them is the importance of relaxing the eyes by being in different light frequencies—adapting to light and adapting to dark. Everybody wears sunglasses, which prevents us from adjusting to the light; in fact, rather than adapt to the light we escape it. We also don't have darkness because in most areas city lights make it impossible. Having so much light at night doesn't allow us to widen the pupils enough to adapt to the dark.

Looking at details is also very important. The macula of the retina, which is only a percent and a half of the total photoreceptor fields, depends on it. As people age, however, they gradually lose the tendency, developed at eight weeks, to be curious and look at details. In addition, in this information age we learn to read not letter by letter or word by word, but paragraph by paragraph in order to digest vast amounts of information. The price we pay for this reading style is that we stop looking at details. As a result, we can suffer from macular degeneration, which is very common.

We also need to look at a distance. Today, many people sit for long periods of time staring at computer monitors rather than using enough distance vision. Our ancestors, by contrast, looked at distant forests to see if animals were around to hunt, and since they did not have weather reports they looked far away at the sky. People who today live in forests, like the indigenous tribes of Brazil, still have amazing vision, as do Bedouins, known to have better than 20/20 vision. The Maori people of New Zealand don't even have the concept of nearsightedness. To compensate for the long periods of time we spend looking at things close up, we need to practice looking at a distance.

Another important principle addressed by my exercises is the use of peripheral vision. The many hours a day we spend looking centrally at our laptop screens, tablets, e-readers, and smartphones have rendered peripheral vision irrelevant. But it was relevant and practiced naturally in the past because people had to look to the sides to avoid danger. Modern-day use of peripheral vision can be reintroduced through eye exercises.

An additional principle to be more aware of is balanced use of the two eyes. Many people have one eye that sees better than the other, and they favor that eye, avoiding use of the one that doesn't see well. We need to stop doing that.

Other principles addressed by the exercises are balanced use within each eye, body-eye coordination, and getting more blood flow to the eyes. I'll give you an exercise that can be done at home. For about two or three minutes, massage your skull from the bottom to the top creating as much separation between the skull and scalp as possible. When you separate the skull and scalp, much more blood flows there.

That is great to do for relaxation too.

Yes. Another good exercise for increasing blood flow to the eyes is to rub your hands together then put them around your eye orbits and visualize seeing complete darkness. As you do this, don't put pressure on your cheekbones. Rest your elbows on a pillow; we have a palming stick to put the elbows on. Keep your shoulders relaxed. Relax your eyes, visualizing them as soft, warm, and floating. Visualize more and more fluid flowing into the eyes. Do this for six minutes.

Practicing these exercises based on the nine principles is the way I've cured myself from blindness, and the way all people can improve their vision and sometimes overcome major vision problems. I used to have 1 percent vision, and now I have 70 percent vision. But this improvement took dedication. People need to understand that either they have to spend time doing physical therapy for their eyes or they're going to spend time at the doctor's office.

I want to create a revolution in eye care because most ophthalmologists tell us our vision can't be improved, yet I've improved my vision greatly by doing these exercises. If you wear glasses, you can get rid of them. If you're forty and read with glasses, you can do the eye exercises to strengthen your eyes just as when you're forty you can do stretches to avoid getting arthritis. We need to work on the body. On its own, it may become stiff because of the type of life we lead.

When you started doing the eye exercises at seventeen, did you think you were going to heal? Did you think you were going to regain your vision? What were you thinking?

I used to read Braille, and I was a son of deaf parents. I admired my parents. They traveled all over Europe being deaf and came to America. My mother was the top actress of the deaf people in Israel. My father was the champion of chess in the deaf club in Israel for several years, and he's in his nineties now. Despite their success, I never liked the idea of being handicapped. I yearned to see. I dreamed about a surgery that would save my sight after the failure of the first five. After a while, the scientific understanding about my situation changed and the doctors started to understand my surgeries were performed poorly and too late to help me develop my vision as an infant. My children's cataracts were removed when they were two weeks old, so when they were eight weeks old they could see the environment around them with contact lenses. They had 20 or 30 percent vision, which ophthalmologists were happy with. But after doing the eye exercises they now have 100 percent vision.

Just as I changed the situation for my children, so am I changing the situation for many other children. My goal is to get people to see better in the beginning.

My work is not only about vision, however; I also do bodywork. We work with people who are in wheelchairs due to muscular dystrophy or multiple sclerosis, and help them walk.

What are the main things you do to help people walk?

First we work on the secondary problem, which has to do with the paralysis. Most paralysis is secondary to the original problem. For instance, with multiple sclerosis you have a drop foot because you don't have strength in your calf anymore. It's not going to put you in a wheelchair. It's going to make you limp, but the tension in your hip joint, neck, and back will make it impossible for you to walk.

One woman told me she had been in a wheelchair for the last twelve years and now cannot write. I found out that being in a wheelchair had made her arms stiff. People in wheelchairs generally don't use their muscles fully, especially to move to the side or backward, or to extend. The resulting stiffness causes great damage. When I loosened this woman up, put her on the floor, and got her to stretch, she could write. When we get muscles that never worked to work, there's progress.

The next thing we do is focus on what can work. There are six hundred muscles in the body, but most people use only fifty. As a result, the connective tissue hardens around joints, making mobility difficult for most people. I teach people who are paralyzed to use the paralyzed areas. Physical therapists tell their patients to do things—such as learn to drive, write, or wash dishes—with their stronger limbs or other body parts. But this leads to more imbalance of the body. By contrast, I teach people to work with the weak areas. Some have seen as much as a 60 or 65 percent improvement.

How is the brain involved in this process?

When connective tissue begins hardening around joints from not fully using our bodies, the idea of decreased usage gets imprinted in the brain. If we start to teach the brain that we need to work more muscles to take the load off our overused muscles, we loosen those muscles, which then begin working better for us.

Let me show you how simple it is to change your functions. Rotate your head in both directions, breathing deeply and slowly. Now rub your hands together while still rotating your head. Then hold your head with your hands and rotate it a few times without the help of your neck muscles.

Taking your hands away, see how easy it is to move your head. If it feels lighter and it means you're really relaxed.

Next close your eyes and visualize rotating your head in both directions. Then, with your eyes closed, visualize your head going all the way to the ceiling and your shoulders moving to opposite sides of the room, as if you were expanding. Now move your head again and see how it feels. Tap on your abdomen and say, "Center, center, center, center, center." Now move your head and see how it feels.

Most people wonder why their head moves more easily after tapping on the belly. It's because they woke up the real center of the body, which is in the navel. The center of the body is not in your chest, where you have a lot of emotions, and it's not in your neck, which holds your head, heavy as it is with thoughts. When you tap your abdomen, the true center of the body, you loosen up your neck.

Would you explain your views on the relationship between clients and practitioners?

Clients and practitioners need to have a partnership. When I see clients, I feel that my forty-five years of experience working is only the starting point. Through massage, I communicate with their condition and develop the touch that addresses their needs, not the touch that you learn in school. Clients learn from me what movements they need to do and tell me what feels best for them. So there's much life in the sessions. That's how we can regenerate bones, muscles, and nerves that work together.

If we just rely on practitioners, what happens?

Practitioners know how to fix symptoms, but then clients will get other ones. Medicine is very good as a patch approach. If something is wrong, doctors remove it. They give medication that's wonderful for some cases and has side effects in others. But this is not a long-term successful approach.

To embark on a long-term successful approach, it's necessary to find a doctor we want to work with and a way that we want to work on ourselves.

For that, we may have to change some of our commonly held beliefs. For example, people believe that eyesight cannot be improved while my message is that it can and it's possible to get rid of glasses. I also think that about 65 percent of people in wheelchairs should not have to use them—that we can avoid most wheelchair use with the correct work. It's unfortunate that more people don't think holistically. If we work on our eyes, we'll see better and the only eye problem we'll have in our nineties will be driving our friends to the ophthalmologist's office.

After you started doing the eye exercises, how long did it take to begin regaining vision?

I noticed some improvement the first time I did the exercises, but it took about three months to improve my vision from 1 percent to 4 percent, and then it took me years to improve my vision more and more.

That is realistic. It takes the body a while to adapt to new processes and protocols. But the fact that your vision improved significantly over time by doing the exercises certainly offers inspiration and hope to others with impaired eyesight.

WISDOM TO REMEMBER

Meir Schneider reminds us that because of our modern lifestyle we have stopped adapting our eyes to light and darkness, near and far distances, peripheral vision, and many other principles of good vision. He has created a natural approach to working with the eyes and the body that helps people see and walk again. He also emphasizes that to avoid only treating symptoms, a long-term cooperative approach is needed that requires dedication, time, and patience.

WHAT YOU CAN DO

To get more blood flow to your eyes, for two to three minutes:

• Massage your skull from the bottom to the top and create separation between the skull and scalp.

Alternatively, for six minutes:

• Rub your hands together and put them around your eye orbits. Avoid putting pressure on your cheekbones or elevating your shoulders, and rest your elbows on something comfortable like a pillow.

• Visualize seeing complete darkness.

• Visualize your eyes as soft, warm, and floating.

• Visualize more and more fluid flowing into your eyes.

To help maintain good kinesthetic awareness, and avoid developing stiffness in the spine, and overcome immobility associated with physical issues such as paralysis and multiple sclerosis, practice this exercise:

• Rotate your head in both directions, breathing deeply and slowly.

• Rub the palms of your hands together while your head is still rotating. Hold your head with your hands and rotate it a few times without the help of your neck muscles.

• Take your hands away, and see how easy it is to move your head.

• Close your eyes and visualize your head rotating in both directions.

• Visualize your head going up to the ceiling and your shoulders moving to opposite sides of the room, as if you were expanding.

- Move your head again and see how it feels.

- Tap on your abdomen and say, "Center, center, center, center, center."

- Move your head and see how it feels now that you woke up the real center of your body, in the navel, which loosens up the head.

CHAPTER 9

The Hormone Balancing Act

THE TRUTH ABOUT ADHD, WEIGHT LOSS, FIBROMYALGIA, AND ANXIETY

With

MICHAEL PLATT, MD

"Next to the promulgation of the truth, the best thing I can conceive that man can do is the public recantation of an error."

—Lord Joseph Lister

Michael Platt, MD, of Platt Wellness Center, was involved in internal medicine from 1972 to 2009. He attended New York Medical College and did his internship and residency at Washington Hospital Center in Washington, DC. Well known for his books *The Miracle of Bioidentical Hormones* and *Adrenaline Dominance*, he has a unique approach to helping people with ADHD, weight challenges, fibromyalgia, anxiety, menopause, migraines, osteoporosis, and restless leg syndrome, among other conditions. From Dr. Platt, I learned the true nature of service: being so passionate about assisting others that one is willing to put one's career and name on the line.

Dr. Platt, would you tell a story about somebody you have helped heal beyond the normal for their situation.

A forty-seven-year old man came to see me complaining of severe fibromyalgia, with a lot of acute muscle aches and pains and a condition called cyclical vomiting syndrome. He was vomiting every morning; as a child had vomited every time he got excited, and couldn't stop, resulting in hospitalization. There's only one cause for this kind of vomiting—excess adrenaline. And excess adrenaline is also the cause of fibromyalgia.

Part of dealing with excess adrenaline is to use another hormone called progesterone in cream form. I put some on his arm, and about five minutes later he declared, "Doc, in my entire life I have never felt this good." It's been almost six years since he came into my office, and he has not had one episode of vomiting since.

This is an account he wrote shortly after I started treating him:

> I first came to Dr. Platt a year and a half ago. I had been on a nine-month merry-go-round of treatments, tests, and scans, all to no avail. Some $118,000 later, an entire staff of doctors could not tell me what was wrong with me. I was suffering from fibromyalgia.... Every single inch of my body hurt. I could not get out of bed in the morning without extreme pain. When I opened Dr. Platt's book *The Miracle of Bio-Identical Hormones*, I found all of my life's agonies described....
>
> I had just lost my job due in part to all these symptoms. My new bride of a year and a half was packing her bags, and frankly I was seriously considering jumping off a bridge. I now know that my adrenal glands are very active, and a CT scan showed me that my adrenal glands are three times larger than the average person's. After reading chapter 15, I also realized that I have ADHD.... The effect that adrenaline has on so many parts of the body simply amazes me—how it affects hypoglycemia and blood sugar.... Adrenaline was killing me.
>
> My wife and I made an appointment to see Dr. Platt.... My mood swings were out of control at this point. Like a clock's pendulum going tick-tock-tick-tock, mine was going aggression-depression-aggression-

depression…. "Do you want all this to go away?" Dr. Platt asked me in the most sincere way, like he just fixed people's lives every day…. He took progesterone cream and spread it down the length of my forearm…. Five minutes or so passed. He asked, "How do you feel?" The first thing that came to mind was what I was not feeling…. I was calm. I was sitting still, perfectly still….

ADHD is a hyperactivity disorder. This comes from too much adrenaline. Too much adrenaline attaching to over 15 million neuroreceptors in the brain equals aggression. My life has always been a battle to calm the aggression…. He put that cream on my arm, and every single symptom was gone….

Dr. Platt…questions the ideas of practitioners who treat the symptoms of disease, not the underlying problem…. The understanding this man has of bioidentical hormones and the human body's reaction to hormone imbalance is astounding…. This man saved my life…. I have a quality of life that thirty years of medical treatment and antidepressants could not give me.

What people sometimes fail to realize is that hormones control every system in the body. Balancing hormones can bring about miraculous life changes in people, as reflected in the title of my first book, *The Miracle of Bioidentical Hormones.* Such transformations are really not miracles, but can be such exceptional improvements that they seem miraculous. Adrenaline is a powerful hormone, which in the old days the body only produced when people were in danger—and thus it's known as the fight-or-flight hormone. Nowadays, some people are producing adrenaline all day and night without being in danger, so it's obviously for a different reason. If we can discover why they're producing adrenaline, we can effect big changes in their lives.

Another patient who experienced a dramatic change was also forty-seven and weighed over four hundred pounds when he first came to see me. Hormones control weight, and people who lose weight usually gain it all back unless the underlying cause is treated. I put this man on a program based on the reason why his body was producing fat, and he eventually got down to a waist size of thirty-two inches from a waist size of fifty some-thing. This man never had a date in his life, but after he lost the weight he started dating, became engaged, and is now married with children.

Would you share more about what he went through before seeing you and what he tried to do?

Hoping to lose weight, he had seen probably a hundred different doctors, and every one of them advised, "Diet and exercise." When he tried follow-ing their suggestions, they all said the same thing: "You're still eating too much." This reflects the mindset of most physicians in our medical system. When doctors see somebody who's overweight, they think they're eating too much. But when I see somebody who's overweight I know their hor-mones are out of balance.

In many overweight people, adrenaline is produced day and night to raise the sugar level to feed the brain. It doesn't matter whether they're eat-ing sugar or whether the body is producing sugar. If it's not burned up, all the extra sugar gets stored as fat in the fat cells.

Then as people produce adrenaline, which creates stress, their bodies re-spond by producing cortisol, which raises the sugar level through different mechanisms. Now these people have two hormones making sugar, both stimulating insulin, which leads to fat around the middle. These are the people who toss and turn at night, who have restless leg syndrome, grind their teeth at night, or get up at night to urinate—all symptoms related to excess adrenaline, the hormone that is possibly the number one cause for weight gain.

Just about everyone has stress. How do the body's responses to it differ from one person to another?

You're right. There are a lot of medical conditions related to excess adren-aline. Adrenaline is an anger hormone, and internalizing anger is probably the number one cause of depression. Excess adrenaline is also likely the only cause of anxiety. Unfortunately, very few doctors ever see it because they are accustomed to giving out "Band-Aids." Adrenaline affects different people in different ways. Some people keep a lot of tension in their necks and shoulders, which is the cause of tinnitus, or ringing in the ears, because the muscles are cutting off circulation to the inner ears.

In my book *Adrenaline Dominance*, I talk about the good, the bad, and the ugly with regard to how adrenaline affects the body. The only condition I put in the good section is attention deficit hyperactivity disorder (AD-HD), which is widely misinterpreted in today's world. People think of AD-HD as being a learning disorder, but instead it is an interest disorder. People with ADHD have no trouble focusing if they're interested. If they're not interested, they will not focus because they've become distracted. Some of the most intelligent, successful, creative people in the world have AD-HD. Creative people have the most adrenaline. You only see bed-wetting in creative children. Mothers who vomit throughout their pregnancies are creative women. Adrenaline is a very interesting hormone that people don't sufficiently discuss or understand.

What's the best thing a person with some of those symptoms can do?

First they need to recognize that they're dealing with excess adrenaline. Next they have to think about why they have excess adrenaline. Besides responding to danger, the only other reason the body produces adrenaline is to raise the sugar level for the brain. But if people give the brain the fuel it needs then the body doesn't have to produce adrenaline.

One way to keep the adrenaline level down is to avoid hypoglycemia, low blood sugar. Whenever insulin goes up, blood sugar goes down. Every time that happens the body produces adrenaline. The primary way to protect against low blood sugar is by applying the hormone progesterone in cream form. Progesterone blocks insulin so people never get sleepy in the afternoon when the insulin level is highest, they don't get sleepy after eating, and they don't get sleepy in a car.

Another way to deal with excess adrenaline is to provide the brain with the right kind of foods. Green vegetables are the perfect sugar for the brain because they don't produce any insulin—they are not glycemic. By contrast, candy, which is the same sugar, glucose, is highly glycemic and produces a lot of insulin. As soon as you eat candy, you get an outpouring of insulin, the sugar level goes down, and the sugar never gets to the brain. The other fuel that the brain uses is ketones, or ketone bodies. The best source of ketones is coconut oil, or what is called MCT (medium-chain triglyceride) oil. If people eat correctly and use progesterone cream, the problem of excess adrenaline goes away. That man who lost so much weight was on progesterone, which blocks insulin, the number one hormone that creates fat.

You mentioned that doctors are trained to put a Band-Aid on rather than treat the underlying causes of diseases. Would you share more about that and your approach to being a doctor?

We don't have a good medical system, primarily because it is controlled by the pharmaceutical industry. This is a big reason why doctors in medical school, internship, and residency programs are not taught the causation of illness. All they are really taught is that if someone has a problem they should take a drug for it. Not only do these drug companies control what doctors learn, they also control the FDA and the medical boards. That's why a lot of progress in medicine has been impeded by the FDA and the medical boards. I help people understand how their bodies operate and how they can fix them. The United States has the highest incidence of diabetes, strokes, heart attacks, cancer, and other diseases. Yet people think we have a good medical system. We have great surgeons but not great medicine.

On your website you also refer to about one hundred thousand people dying from medicine a year. What is that about?

Over one hundred thousand people a year die from prescription medications, which is called iatrogenic disease. Iatrogenic diseases are the third leading cause of death now, after cancer and heart disease. I have tried to change health care in this country by pointing out different ways of approaching it, but it's hard to change people's minds.

Whose minds do we need to change?

We need to make doctors realize there are alternatives. Diabetes is usually an easy condition to get rid of. So is hypertension. But drugs that doctors give to lower cholesterol should never be used because cholesterol is not the enemy. In fact, people with the highest cholesterol have the greatest longevity. Our mindset is drugs. Doctors try to lower the patient's cholesterol, lower their blood sugar, and lower their blood pressure, thinking they're helping the patient, but they're hurting the patient. All they need to do is treat the underlying reason for the blood pressure elevation. Insulin and adrenaline are the two hormones that raise blood pressure, and their levels are easy to control.

Give us a tip for people with diabetes or those who need to lower their insulin levels so they can get off drugs.

There are actually three different types of diabetes. Type 1 diabetics are people who don't have any insulin, and they need insulin. Type 2 diabetics, the most common group, are people who usually have a lot of insulin but are insulin resistant. Type 3 diabetics have resistance to insulin in the brain—that is, the brain can't get sugar into the brain cells. This is probably the number one predisposing factor to Alzheimer's disease. Currently, the drug of choice for Alzheimer's is coconut oil, which converts to ketones, which, in turn, do not need insulin to get into the brain cells. So coconut oil is actually good for any neurodegenerative type of disease.

When it comes to type 2 diabetes, if you know that insulin is perhaps the problem then putting the person on something like progesterone, which blocks the effects of insulin, can usually get them off their medications. I never had any diabetic patients whom I was not able to get off medications except some type 1 diabetics. But even some of those I was able to get off medications because they had been mistakenly put on insulin.

What can most people do to ensure their health and longevity that they may not already be doing?

People need to be careful about what they're eating. Long ago Hippocrates talked about the importance of food for health. People should avoid refined sugars and other foods they know are not healthy, such as genetically modified foods and foods with rBST, a hormone to stimulate milk production in cows—a carcinogen that, consequently, also goes into cheese and yogurt. Unfortunately, the United States is one of the few countries that allows genetically modified foods and about the only country that allows rBST.

People also need to be careful about medications. Drugs are, for the most part, toxic. There is only one drug I know of that actually cures a disease—hepatitis C. They put a price tag of $85,000 on it for a three-month supply when it probably costs $20 to manufacture.

How would you determine if a particular doctor is the right one to visit?

In a perfect world, people would go to a doctor who practiced what's called functional medicine, which treats the causation of illness. But rarely do even functional medicine doctors know much about adrenaline or hormones. One of the big problems in medicine is that doctors treat lab tests, not patients. When it comes to hormones, you can never go wrong treating a patient, but you can go awfully wrong treating a lab test about hormones because hormones change daily, weekly, and monthly. I wrote books to put people in charge of their health so they won't have to rely on doctors so much.

Another problem is that there is no preventive medicine in this country. Flu shots do not prevent the flu; they cause it. Similarly, we both know that mammograms do not prevent breast cancer, but the radiation can actually exacerbate cancer or cause it, while progesterone cream prevents breast cancer, as do high doses of vitamin D.

Do you recommend people consult with a doctor before using progesterone cream? Is it possible to absorb too much of it?

Progesterone is a very safe hormone. Progesterone cream, not the pill, blocks the three most toxic hormones in the body —estrogen, insulin, and adrenaline. A lot of doctors think it's a woman's hormone, but men and women have identical hormones. Progesterone is also wonderful for babies who have colic. It gets rid of colic in about three minutes because colic is an anxiety caused by adrenaline, as is the "terrible twos." Progesterone can help with bed-wetting as well, which is caused by adrenaline. Progesterone can get rid of ADHD in about twenty-four hours. People may wonder if it's dangerous to give a child hormones, but when babies are in the womb they are exposed to high levels of progesterone; it's the hormone that allows their brains to develop, so it's not a bad hormone to give to children. It is important to note that the exact strength of progesterone cream needs to be 5% in order to block adrenaline and insulin, which is available on my website without the need for a prescription. The question is, can people do such treatments on their own. They probably can, but if they have questions they could always get in touch with my office.

I'd like to highlight a hopeful comment that you made on your website—that all the treatments we call miracles would one day become routine.

WISDOM TO REMEMBER

In a medical system that often focuses on treating lab results with drugs, Dr. Platt stands out by concentrating on the underlying causes of physical conditions.

If you or anyone you know has experienced any of the following symptoms, Dr. Platt suggests it is likely due to excess adrenaline:

- Muscle aches and pains

- Excessive vomiting

- Bed-wetting and needing to pee a lot at night

- Weight gain

- Sleeplessness

- Restless leg syndrome
- Grinding teeth while sleeping
- Feeling sleepy from 3:00 to 4:00 p.m.
- Anger
- Depression
- Anxiety
- Neck tension
- Tinnitus (ringing in the ears)
- Hypoglycemia
- Fibromyalgia
- ADHD
- Breast cancer
- Colic

WHAT YOU CAN DO

If you suffer from any of the above conditions:

- Consider getting a progesterone cream to rub on your forearm.
- Eat lots of green vegetables.
- Add coconut oil or an MCT (medium-chain triglyceride oil) to your diet.

- Avoid genetically modified foods.

- Avoid refined sugars.

To help heal diabetes and Alzheimer's disease:

- Add coconut oil to your diet.

To help heal breast cancer:

- Add more vitamin D to your diet.

PART IV

Sound, Light, Air, Energy, and Healing

CHAPTER 10

Healing with Your Voice
A Hepatitis C Miracle

With
Tryshe Dhevney

"I know why the caged bird sings."

—Maya Angelou

While on a five-week road trip through the United States, I stopped at a yoga studio in Tucson to practice restorative yoga. To my surprise, there was a beautiful woman named Tryshe Dhevney with bright red hair sitting with singing bowls around her. She explained that she had been given a year to live until she started toning and playing singing bowls. Now she has told her story in her book *Sound Shifting*, and she travels around the country with ten to twenty bowls, sharing her method of sound healing.

Tryshe, you were a major inspiration for this book about healing. I love your book, *Sound Shifting*, which is also the name of your business. You've continued to be a specialist in sound healing. Please share the story of your health journey.

It was a very circuitous journey. In the beginning, I had no symptoms of disease, per se, except that I felt stressed and exhausted. At the time, I was working with young people as an artistic director of an acting company. So I thought, *Who wouldn't be exhausted doing this kind of work?* I paid no attention to my condition until I moved to Tucson, where I got married and then had a routine checkup. My physician made the diagnosis, declaring, "It's showing up that your liver is compromised and you have hepatitis C."

It was 1998 and the disease had just been named. Not knowing much about it, I assumed it was something like the flu and was not too concerned. But later a friend had a strong reaction to the news and exclaimed, "Oh my God, this is serious."

I called the doctor back and asked, "What do I do?"

And she answered, "There really isn't anything we can do, but let me refer you to a team of doctors."

At the time, there was a chemical therapy called interferon that doctors were exploring. The team gave me the option of trying it; but instead I opted to go the route of alternative medicine. I changed my diet. I had acupuncture. I did qigong. I went to a psychic surgeon. I worked with a range of healers, all while my viral load got increasingly higher and the virus mutated. One team member left a message on my answering machine stating that they had exhausted all possible treatment options and suggesting I get my affairs in order.

Then I sought the opinion of another doctor, who said, "Indeed, this is serious. Let's see about putting you on interferon." It was at that moment, I believe, that my healing began, because I let go.

How was the experience of being sick up to that point?

I had little or no attunement to what was going on in my body. I had overcompensated so skillfully that I assumed my symptoms were the result of regular stress and I would just pull up my bootstraps and carry on—drink a little more green tea. In fact, I had never not been ill. Hepatitis C mutates in the body and remains dormant for years—in my case, about thirty years. Within two days of putting me on an interferon-ribavirin combination that I injected into my body, the doctor noticed my immune system was compromised and started lowering my dose, though he never told me why until later.

Meanwhile, I went to a gem show where a vendor selling gorgeous Tibetan singing bowls showed me how to play one, and I spontaneously broke into song. Time seemed to stop. I felt glorious, full of life. I bought the bowl and played it regularly, enjoying the experience but not thinking that it offered a potential for healing. I had accepted that I was dying.

Soon after, I shared a tool with my young acting students that I thought helped access deeper authenticity in their work, called chakra tones. I was given them in the 1970s when a Sufi order came to our Omega Theater Company. I saw extraordinary transformation in these young people and thought, *I have nothing to lose. Let me start to do these tones.* Doing them gave me the feeling of being centered no matter what was going on around me.

After three months, my doctor disclosed, "We're guardedly optimistic. We're not too sure what happened, but we can't find any virus in your body." I thought, *Wow, I wonder if that had anything to do with the exposure to sound?* I still continued doing the toning because it felt good. And the doctor kept testing me, but only every nine months.

Two years after the virus had disappeared the nurse explained why the doctor was so mystified by my situation. She told me, "You don't have a genotype that would have responded to interferon, so there's no medical reason for you to be well." And then I knew it was due to sound. That was the defining moment for me.

After that, I started to read as much research about the effects of sound as possible. One pivotal researcher, Fabian Maman, was exploring the effects of instruments—piano, horn, drum, guitar—which had no notable impact on cell structure. Later he found that the sound of the voice destabilized cancer cells and revitalized normal cells, making the cancer disappear. He tested this on several women with various tumors and found that their masses disintegrated, including that of one woman who'd had surgery, though she had been part of a study using toning for a half hour a day for months. When they opened her up and found that her mass was beginning to disintegrate, they became convinced that toning not only was helping to revitalize cells but was balancing endocrine systems, changing the way the brain worked, lowering blood pressure, and reducing stress, which turned out to be the key element in my healing.

The body knows how to heal; I just didn't know how to get out of the way. Because I had the expectation that I was sick, my thoughts were preventing my healing. In a sense, I was blessed with cluelessness. I didn't know it was possible to become healthy after being diagnosed with hepatitis C and told I had a year to live.

How would you recommend that others get the mind out of the way so it doesn't interrupt their healing?

Sound makes it possible for us to be grounded in the moment while expanding our awareness. Our brains can't comprehend what that is. When we make a simple sound, the body is in the present moment. There is no way you can start to manipulate cells at that point. Sound reawakens the body's natural frequency, restoring harmony to the whole organism.

Making a tone overrides our previous perception of who we are in time and space. Old stories collected over the years or that have been imprinted on us between ages two and five have rearranged the way our brains gather and sequence data. Working with sound overrides those old programs and restores the natural resonance of our bodies. It resequences the brain and creates new neural networks that enable us to access the crystalline core of our beings, where we intuitively know how to navigate life's situations. Healing isn't about eradicating symptoms; it is about restoring resonance.

Trying to eradicate symptoms creates a frequency of illness. Sound allows us to release what we imagine is happening and let our bodies do what they are designed to do.

What is the difference between curing and healing?

Curing is the eradication of symptoms. Healing is the restoration of resonance and harmony to the body, even if it's getting ready to transition. In my case, the symptoms were eradicated because I believed I was not yet ready to leave this planet, that I still had work to do. If it had been my time to transition, that would have been my exit strategy. The restoration of resonance would have ensured that I wasn't carrying a boatload of negativity—fear, resistance, smallness, density, and stress—with me so I could exit with a harmonious body and soul.

In your book, you say you do not consider your transformation to be a miracle. Would you explain what that means.

The doctor called me his miracle girl, but I said, "It's not a miracle. I really think we're onto something here." However, he wasn't able to embrace the idea of tone restoring resonance and harmony to the body. Fortunately, I am working with young doctors in the Integrative Wellness Institute at the University of Arizona who are being exposed to energy medicine and vibrational medicine, which is broadening their sense of healing so that they are not just looking at curing but at the whole human structure—body, mind, spirit.

When my doctor looks at my transformation as an anomaly, I argue, though not out loud, that we are all equipped with the ability to heal this way. It's just that we don't know how to allow it to happen. The remedy is on the tips of our tongues—breathing—and in the sounds we make in the sea of vibration in which we live. When we are in harmony with all that is, we are in a state of nonresistance. That is the healing state.

Beautiful. It seems what you are saying is that we all have the potential to heal ourselves with the sounds that come from our own bodies.

Absolutely. Where it becomes tricky is how we perceive ourselves. If we adhere to a long-held assumption of smallness, we silence our voices and don't allow ourselves to breathe. In that state, we cannot access the overall resonance and spectrum of overtones available to us and so the sound we produce is limited. I teach people how to open up, breathe deeper, and project sounds from the depth of their bodies out to the universe. Most will start to make sound that is like an arm growing out increasingly further, but then stop. Often they have such limiting thoughts as *I've said enough, I'm too loud,* or *I'm interrupting* related to how they perceive themselves.

Opening up sound energizes the breath and oxygenates the body whether we are restoring resonance intentionally or not. In doing this, our voices become a meditation, a blessing, and a gift to the world. Then we are not putting forth the dissonance, caution, and smallness but instead continuously opening to larger perspectives and realms.

I do a lot of chanting, and I find that when I am being expansive in myself and feeling confident the sound is fuller and smoother. It's very weak or choppy or quiet when I am in a more contracted state.

Exactly. The ancient Vedics talked about sound as expressing the fullness of our beings. When we are thinking small, when we are perceiving ourselves as less than, we're not experiencing the fullness of our beings. We may have an idea that we want to be doing something more exciting or creative, but we can't because it doesn't happen in the brain. It occurs in the full body harmonic—the pleroma, as it is called in the Vedic tradition. Experiencing the fullness of being allows us to be in touch with the soul of our sound, the soul of life itself.

As someone familiar with the relationship between yogic tradition and healthy living, could you comment on why a lot of people get sick even when they feel like they've been doing a lot to support their health.

Truth be told, there was a period in my life when I did not eat healthy foods, drank too much, and did not have a balanced lifestyle. I was in recovery for thirty-six years. After getting sober, I wasn't necessarily a good eater and didn't exercise enough. It wasn't until I became ill that I began paying attention to this extraordinary vehicle I'm in. The solution was, ironically, letting go and being willing to *not* try to fix it.

When people are doing many things to be well, they are operating under the assumption that they're not well. The work with sound brings us back to knowing that we are at our cores whole, vibrant, creative, passionate, and masterful in everything we do, with knowledge of how to live in this world. That's our birthright.

Trying to be well may entail different practices for different people—and that's fine. It's really about listening to our personal preferences. Herein lies the gift that happens with sound as we have conversations with our bodies; our bodies tell us, "This activity feels good. This kind of food feels good." I don't eat bad food anymore because my body won't tolerate it. When I do, it says, "Let's help you understand what this does."

I did an experiment recently. Since my body is healthier than it used to be, and not so reactive to my food allergies, I decided to try a little of those foods. But I felt awful, and asserted, "Experiment over."

It's a journey, isn't it? It's not about the destination. We're on a journey through the harmonics of being. We're learning about our bodies and how to rewire them. I found that I could reconstruct my body through sound and breath because our sound energizes the breath. These are the two elements that clear the head, which is operating according to old programs. The old self-perceptions will always be there, but they recede so they're no longer dominant. Our response will now be: "Tell the truth. Open the heart. Make sound. Don't be afraid."

A couple of years ago I had an opportunity to open a Sounds True conference with a heart-centered song. I had no idea what I was going to do. I just breathed, dropped into my heart, and opened my voice. What came out was something I couldn't have anticipated—an incredible experience. At one point, I gazed out at the thousands of faces and felt that we were all part of the fabric of sound and in a place of complete authenticity. If I had tried to plan that, I might have had much smaller energy, but I knew I had to risk meeting myself in this way.

Every day I have an opportunity to reach beyond my perceptions through sound and toning. When we make sounds, we invoke affirmations, which I call seeds of transformation. This occurs because we're creating a combined alpha theta brain state, a highly suggestible fertile ground where we are open to new ideas. After I make a sound, I will grab one of those seeds of transformation and affirm it out loud. Then I'll feel it move through my entire body, down to my toes. It takes root in the Gaia, the earth, because that is my true nature, that is *our* true nature.

Thank you for that. What is something readers could do right now to start on the journey of allowing sound to help them be expansive and present?

That state is only a breath away. Just open your mouth a couple of fingers wide. The more we open, the more breath and resonance we have. I invite people to make the sound "Aaahhh," the sound of the heart chakra. It activates what is called the *siddhi* consciousness, the consciousness of the higher mind, our awakened self. Physiologically it also lowers blood pressure, reduces stress, and stimulates immune function.

Somebody who can't comfortably do an open tone can always hum, "Mmmmm," a straight tone. Or they can make a nonsensical sound—anything that does not have them singing a song. You want to just roam, go on a journey of awakening.

Another great way to open up the gateway of sound is to wake up in the morning and glide—start really low, go higher in pitch, then come back down. Doing that a few times wakes the body up and stimulates the endocrine glands and chakras. To do something more refined, work with the chakra tones.

Do you have any final thoughts you would like to share?

To achieve healing, I would recommend concentrating on the state of nonresistance. Nonresistance allows our bodies to do what they are designed to do. It also restores our access to who we truly are at a vibratory, subatomic level. Sound is uniquely designed to shift us into a state of nonresistance and restore balance.

A little exercise to attain nonresistance is to let your jaw fall and belly soften when you are feeling afraid or tight. Then breathe and make the sound "Aaahhh."

I just started going to Toastmasters. One of the most common things I've noticed is that people need to relax their jaws to better articulate sound.

Yes, and doing that also makes it more authentic. There are so many layers to sound, especially when we are speaking. If we're not breathing well, our audiences can't connect and breathe with us, so they fall asleep or get agitated. The more relaxed we are and speak from our hearts, the more expansive and harmonious we feel, as do others around us.

WISDOM TO REMEMBER

Initially, Tryshe Dhevney did not know she had hepatitis C or that her daily practice of toning was healing her. It enabled her to be in a state of nonresistance, where sound was bypassing her mind, grounding her, expanding her awareness, and returning her to a natural state of harmony. This is no miracle, as the body has the potential to heal itself. Having a positive perspective of yourself and not trying to fix yourself are other keys to healing.

WHAT YOU CAN DO

- A simple way to tone is to open your mouth wide and sing "Ahhhh" from your heart.

- In the morning when you wake up, start singing "Ahhhh" at a low pitch, then gliding high and low again, all in one breath.

- When you feel fearful, relax your jaw and soften your belly. Then breathe while making the sound "Aaahhh."

CHAPTER 11

A New Normal
SOUND AND LIGHT HEALING BROKEN BONES

With
GAIL LYNN

"The day science begins to study non-physical phenomena, it will make more progress in one decade than in all the previous centuries of its existence."

—Nikola Tesla

G ail Lynn operates the Life Center in Westminster, Colorado, where she utilizes a unique sound and light healing technology in order to relieve emotional, physical, and environmental trauma. Over five thousand people from all over the United States and eight other countries have visited Gail to be treated in these sound and light chambers. A sonic massage in one of them left me with the same feeling I had after my best meditation experience—light, happy, and free.

I hear that the sound and light technology you use has had major effects on people, sometimes helping them heal beyond what their doctors predicted for their situations. Gail, would you tell us a story about one of those cases.

An eighty-year-old woman with a broken ankle came to the center in a cast and using a walker. I advise people to do one set of three sessions a month for three months to retrain the body. I explain to them that it doesn't work overnight as it takes time to retrain the body from injuries and patterns, but this woman claimed she was going to try it for only three days. Afterward, she said, "Nothing happened. But I'll do what you said and try it for three months." The next time she came in, three weeks later, she didn't have a cast or walker yet said, "Nothing happened, but I'm still going to do more because that's what you advised." She did a second set of sessions and explained, "Nothing happened." Then she came in for her third set of sessions with a tennis shoe on instead of a boot and said, "Nothing happened." That's just three months of progress for an eighty-year-old woman who had a bad ankle break needing screws and other hardware to fix it.

She finished her three months of sessions and went back to her orthopedic surgeon, who confessed, "I don't understand. Your bone density went back to 100 percent. I'm going to take the hardware out six months early." But she still kept telling me, "Nothing happened."

After this, when I would see her name show up on my phone's caller ID phone I wouldn't answer because I was tired of hearing her tell me, "Nothing happened." Then one day I got this message: "Can you call me back? I need to eat crow." I called her back, and she said, "Lots happened." She shared that the doctor told her that twenty-year-old patients don't heal as fast as she did. That's probably one of the funniest stories I have.

Why do you think she didn't notice that anything was happening?

I have no idea. Many times the changes are so subtle that people just float along and don't notice them. I asked her, "Did you tell your doctor you've been treated with sound and light technology?" She replied, "No. He would have thought I was crazy."

Another time a woman came in who'd had headaches every day for ten years. After she did a set of sessions, she said, "Nothing happened." I asked, "Well, how are the headaches?" She didn't have them anymore! She didn't even realize it. Again, sometimes subtle changes happen in response to this sound and light technology and people tell me, "Nothing happened."

I have felt that when people are getting healing treatments of any kind but thinking nothing happened it may mean that they have integrated the changes so fully that their consciousness has been altered and they can't recognize what has happened.

Right! I call it achieving a "new normal."

That's a good way of expressing it. How did you begin working with this technology?

I met the designer of the original technology at a conference in Los Angeles in 2001 while I was involved in a movie project in Hollywood. His talk was so impactful. I told him I'd had migraine headaches for twenty-three years and asked if the sound and light technology would help with them. He replied, "Well, the body doesn't know disease by name." Being a corporate girl, I was black and white. I want a yes or no answer. I thought, *What an idiot. That's not an answer.* At the time, I did not know that the FDA had rules prohibiting natural healers from making health claims about such technology.

Then in 2007 I was experiencing severe cardiovascular stress, as well as asthma and cystic acne. My hair was falling out. I was on thyroid medicine. I was in a downward spiral. I kept running into the designer, so I decided to travel to the Arizona Center to try the technology. I was so out of tune with my body that, at first, I would likely have said, "Nothing happened." But in a few weeks my asthma was gone, I was having fewer migraines, my autonomic nervous system was back in balance, and my cardiovascular stress was better, so clearly something did happen.

In 2008, I did another set of sessions. In 2009, I was almost at the point where I had no medical issues and was feeling so great that I momentarily thought of becoming a practitioner to help others. But being a corporate girl, I told the universe, "I'm not going to get involved with a medical type of business." The universe said, "Oh yes you are!"

The rest of the year was like a bad country song. I lost my dog, my job, my house, and I filed for bankruptcy. I was in another downward spiral. In 2010, I said yes to the universe, announcing, "There's nothing left but to open a sound and light healing center. Okay, fine. I'll do it." Six months later my life was perfect—no more migraines, no more asthma, no more hair falling out, no more cystic acne, no more prescription meds. I started my business with the first-generation model, graduated to the second generation, and have since evolved the technology to produce greater results—and that's how my new design, the Harmonic Egg, was born in 2017. Getting involved with this form of energy healing was definitely my destiny; it's what I was put on the planet to do.

What else helped you transition from having a corporate mindset to being open to this type of energy healing?

I was first introduced to the concepts of energy healing in 1998, while married to a shaman. He helped start me on the path of traveling to places like Peru, Egypt, Indonesia, and Malaysia to learn more about energy healing from different cultural perspectives, though I didn't think I would do it as a career. However, the universe had taken my former identity away through all the hardship I'd experienced, thus I had to start over. It was a blessing in disguise. It wasn't easy, but things worth doing are never easy.

When people come to you doubtful about this type of healing method, how do you get them to become more open to its healing potential?

It depends on their orientation. To those oriented to Western, or allopathic, medicine, I speak the language of the autonomic nervous system; probably fifteen doctors refer patients to me because of this. I explain to each client how vibrations can balance their autonomic nervous system. I tell them how trauma causes disease, that being stuck in fight-or-flight mode makes the nervous system create something undesirable in the body, such as allergies, insomnia, Parkinson's disease, or worse. I mention that three kinds of trauma exist—emotional, physical, and environmental—as the main causes of disease. We have done medical testing, such as heart rate variability testing, pre- and post- urinalysis testing, and blood work analysis, so clients favoring Western medicine can feel comfortable knowing that something here might help them.

And when I get the esoteric, airy-fairy types of clients I talk to them about how this energy healing works with regard to the different dimensions. We use sacred geometry with the sound and light to help activate the pineal gland, increase circulation, and decrease inflammation, so there's also a spiritual aspect to it. It's a brilliant technology.

What is that spiritual aspect?

The spiritual aspect of this technology becomes evident especially when children receive treatments. This may seem farfetched, but they tell me about angels and other beings present during sessions. For instance, a child of about six or seven, who had been born with the hemispheres of her brain out of balance, was having a session while I chatted with her mom on the couch in the room. We left the chamber door open so the child would not be scared, and she called out, "You guys need to close the door because the white being is working on my head."

Another time my sister, who hadn't been able to get pregnant for fifteen years, was in the chamber. She told me afterward that she was a bit scared because there was something in the chamber with her, but explained, "It felt okay, so I didn't jump out." One week after she balanced her autonomic nervous system and was out of fight-or-flight mode, her body was able to tune in to reproduction and not just survival, and now she and her husband have a five-year-old child.

Even if it is not true that those beings exist, I can see how it must have been comforting for them to think of a nonphysical presence supporting their healing process.

I agree. I grew up near Detroit and didn't believe in this stuff prior to having the Life Center and now I'm experiencing firsthand many things I would have judged others for believing.

Also on a spiritual level, I think my intuition has improved from doing sessions in the chamber. For example, I can now feel if there is tension between different aspects of a person and whether it is rooted in emotional, physical, or environmental trauma in their body. It's been interesting to see how I've evolved as a result of using this technology. It's opened me to experiencing greater energy flow. For instance, once when I stated to a client I needed to learn more about Egyptian technologies, lo and behold a woman showed up who had been living in Cairo for thirty years. My motto now is "Ask and you shall receive—and be careful what you ask for." Manifesting what I envision is easier now, and things seem to flow divinely.

Tell us more about how the technology works.

The technology brings together both sound and light in a powerful way in one machine. Interestingly, Edgar Cayce, the "sleeping prophet," wrote in his book *Auras*, "If colors are vibrations of spiritual forces, they should be able to help in healing our deepest and most subtle maladies. Together with music, which is a kindred spiritual force, they form a great hope for therapy of the future." The designer of the first- and second-generation technologies was born in January 1948, three years after Cayce's death, and has the same gifts as Cayce. He can do readings and scan someone's body from 1,200 miles away to see what's going on.

How would you explain the power of the combination of sound and light?

Its power was known by ancient cultures. I'm studying the ancient Egyptians because they used vibration, sound, and light for healing in sarcophagus chambers. Australian Aborigines started doing sound healing with a didgeridoo probably forty thousand years ago. I think sound is more powerful than light, especially the sound in the chamber and the resonance clients bathe in during sessions. We use wood to line the chamber because wood doesn't hold energy or information. We don't use crystals in the chamber because crystals hold information and we don't want anybody to be affected by the energy of others who have been in there. Even the deprivation chambers can hold energy in the water. I feel the vibration of the toxins from that energy needs to be cleared from the water.

The musical instruments we use for each client are based on their symptoms and what they want to work on during the session. For example, drumming can help build the immune system and sometimes helps eliminate anxiety and depression. Piano sounds can help balance the nervous system, while flute sounds can sometimes help with sciatica pain, gout, and anger-related issues.

Can such sounds be produced by people at home by playing instruments, for example?

They can produce some healing sounds at home or listen to them through headphones. We put the whole body inside the chamber and surround the body with instrumental sounds. The result has been described as sound and music on steroids. Immersing the whole body—as opposed to just listening to music through the ears or in a large room where sound dissipates—seems to allow the systems to work in harmony. People familiar with the last part of yoga where you are lying on your back in deep relaxation, or *shavasana,* say the experience in the chamber is like *shavasana* amplified.

Even for those who don't believe in it, it works. One time a man with Parkinson's disease was in the chamber and said, "I don't want to be here. My church sent me and paid for it. I can't wait to tell them it didn't work." He came out; took a step; looked down at his foot, which was no longer shuffling from the Parkinson's; and started to cry with relief. He had not taken a heel to toe step in more than a year.

Have you ever contacted people later to see if the healing was sustained?

Yes, and it was. On the other hand, a Vietnam vet who had been exposed to Agent Orange called. After his first set of sessions, he started walking faster. Initially it took him almost a half hour to get from the parking lot to being positioned in the chamber. The second day it took twenty minutes, and the third day only twelve minutes. He did two sets, after which I advised him to continue retraining the cell memory because cells can go back to what they remembered before. Eventually he went on vacation and stopped, and now he's crashed again and having a hard time moving.

It's essential to explain to people with a chronic condition that they have to continue to retrain the body. Healing is not magic; it takes time for the body to learn new patterns and habits. You don't run a marathon after jogging around the block. You train for months or longer to prepare the body. In healing, you need to give the body time to retrain the cell memory and learn a *new normal*. We can't help people who won't help themselves. I understand that some can't afford to keep coming, but they could at least do something to keep up the energy or come once a month as a commitment to their evolution and healing.

What do you think prevents people from keeping up that energy?

Old habits. If you're going to keep doing the same things you've always done, you're going to get the same results you've always gotten. If you're going to go back to eating at Taco Bell, Arby's, and Kentucky Fried Chicken and drinking seven Diet Pepsis a day, you're not going to keep up that energy.

Emotional changes need to happen as well. If you are going to stay angry with the world and not change your attitude, you most likely will stay unhealthy.

I don't even tell people they have to exercise, but they do have to increase circulation by walking or doing gentle yoga. Personally, I don't go to the gym to work out; instead, I ride or play with my horse six or seven days a week. Many people increase inflammation from working out too hard and too much, and, as we now know, inflammation creates disease. Stress, sugar, and poor eating habits also cause inflammation.

For sessions to have the best chance of succeeding, people can't go back to doing the same things they've always done, especially if they have cancer, which involves a lot of emotional trauma, mutated viruses, or energy blocks. They've got to be willing to let go of old ways. If you understand Chinese medicine, the lungs hold grief, the liver holds anger, and the kidneys hold fear. People have got to be willing to look at what got them to where they are and learn how to change things.

We can release a lot of emotional trauma at a cellular level, which is especially good for PTSD, freeing soldiers from having to relive wars and trauma. After sessions, PTSD sufferers say things like, "I don't feel the monkey is on my back" or "I feel like I left my stuff in the room"—meaning they've found some relief from the issues that were plaguing them.

What most helps people change their habits?

Learning to listen to their bodies because everything's a message. I'll often advise clients to read books that describe messages from the body, like those by Louise Hay, *Feelings Buried Alive Never Die* by Karol K. Truman, or *Who's the Matter with Me?* by Alice Steadman. If a group of people ski down the same mountain and one breaks a neck, another breaks a wrist, another dies, and nothing happens to a fourth, each injury, or lack thereof, is a message from each individual body signaling what needs attention. I also educate people about diet—explaining the disadvantages of eating processed foods and genetically modified foods—and about being exposed to pollution, allergens, and other environmental offenders.

In addition, some of my clients work with trauma therapists, EFT practitioners, DOs, or MDs. They can get some help from these practitioners as well. There's never one solution for everybody. Everyone must find the right combination for themselves. The universe takes care of us by bringing the right people into our lives for healing.

Is there anything else you'd like to share about the sound and light technology, or healing in general?

The technology helped me a great deal on an emotional level. I didn't remember a lot of my childhood because of trauma. The technology helped me let go of that painful "story." Once I helped a woman with a brain injury who did the opposite. She was a psychologist, and she left one day after her session saying, "Thank you very much. This is helping me, but I'm never coming back because I don't know who I would be without my brain injury." She was not willing to change her story and take responsibility for her health.

Many people come in on several prescription drugs. About eighty percent of the symptoms they list in their paperwork are direct side effects of the meds, and they don't realize it. I often refer them to the book entitled

Drug Muggers so they can review the drugs they are on and what they deplete from the body. Most prescription drugs deplete some or many nutrients that need to be replenished to prevent the occurrence of more side effects. For example, all statin drugs deplete CoQ10, a coenzyme that is good for heart health and regulates blood pressure, among other benefits. We need to be aware of what we are putting into our bodies and how it can affect us.

How would you summarize the healing process you offer in one word that can be easily remembered?

The word that comes to mind is *hope*.

That's a very inspirational word. I feel it's possible to create a healing environment within oneself by thinking about and speaking such inspirational words as *hope* that are considered to have a good vibration.

WISDOM TO REMEMBER

Gail Lynn makes it clear that disease can be caused by emotional, physical, or environmental trauma. The Life Center technology can recalibrate our bodies through a combination of light and sound that heals and reduces trauma, and returns cells to their natural resonance. Sometimes it feels like nothing is happening after the sessions because people have already integrated the changes and are experiencing a "new normal."

Gail believed in the technology because of her experience with it. If there is anything about it that you doubt, she advises trying it for yourself and basing your judgement on the results. The ailments in our bodies are often related to emotions with which we struggle. We accelerate our healing when we willingly discard old habits, change our stories, and take more responsibility for our own healing.

WHAT YOU CAN DO

After feeling the effects of emotional, physical, or environmental trauma, you can actively participate in your healing by taking following actions:

- Participate in healing sessions over a long period of time so they have a greater effect and lasting benefits.

- Change your habits so the disease or illness does not return.

- Adopt a healthier diet devoid of processed and genetically altered foods.

- Engage in activities that promote circulation in the body, such as yoga, walking, or gentle exercises.

- Research the side effects of medications you are taking.

- Listen to your body!

CHAPTER 12

The Energy Dance
BIRD FLU FLIES AWAY, AND ADULT LEGS GROW

With

BHAVNA SRIVASTAVA

"Love is a fruit in season at all times, and within reach of every hand."

—Mother Teresa

Bhavna Srivastava, known as the Golden Light Goddess, is a healer, Reiki master, and spiritual teacher. Holding an MBA from New York State University, she works with a group of holistic practitioners at Bhavna's Wellness Group to bring peace and love to people's bodies, minds, hearts, and spirits for holistic healing. In my energy healing sessions with her I have felt uplifted spiritually and enlightened by her wisdom.

Bhavna, would you share your story of how you got into healing, and healed someone beyond what was expected.

At the time, I was in a totally different world, being an MBA with a background in banking and finance. The event that shifted my interest to healing was when my brother, who lives in India, got the bird flu during an epidemic in 2007, when people were dying from it.

He'd gone to a dinner party where he'd eaten chicken and ended up in the hospital in a very bad state, unable to even get up or talk. My brother was a lively person, married, with two boys. He was the type of person who would go out of his way to do anything for others. It was heartbreaking to see him in this condition. The doctors gave up and told my father, "We cannot do anything more for him. Please take him home, do your prayers, and call family members." Then my father called me, crying, and said, "Bhavna, do something."

It takes an hour or two to prepare the discharge papers, so I figured I had only that amount of time in which to turn things around. Therefore, I replied, "Give me some time."

I focused healing energy on my brother for an hour. After that, I received a call from my father saying, "He got up and went to the bathroom."

Everybody in the hospital was shocked because for the past ten days my brother had been bedridden. I thought, *Wow, what happened?* Then instead of discharging him they readmitted him, saying, "We will see what's going on." Today he's healthy, happy, and living with his family in India.

That experience made me think that I have gifts for healing, for which I credit the Divine. I also have had experiences with others that reinforced my commitment to the healing profession and made me realize how much I love and desire to help all people— feelings that had been awakened by the incident with my brother.

At the time, you were involved with finance. When your father called and said, "Do something," how did you know what to do, and what did you actually do?

Even though I was in finance, I was already a Reiki master but used those skills only for personal stress reduction and to help friends manage stress. My logical brain was much more active than my creative brain. But when my father said, "Do something," I knew there was nothing else to do but try to use my healing skills to help my brother. What I did was not just Reiki but a combination of methods: I chanted, I prayed, and I used healing energies.

Did you know before you started working on your brother that you were going to make a difference?

I was very confident, somehow. I felt I had strength. I have a little temple in my house, which I made. I sat in front of the temple with my brother's picture, and things just moved.

Somebody reading this might say, "Oh maybe that was just a fluke." Have you been able to help heal other people who had received a terminal diagnosis?

Yes. Lots of times I've helped people in situations such as alcohol addiction, where doctors pronounced they wouldn't live. I worked on them, and they lived.

One person had primary lymphedema on her left side, causing her left leg to be bigger than her right one. She had gone through surgeries, acupuncture, and other treatments without success, and the doctor proclaimed she would just have to live with one bigger leg. Now, after working on her over three years, I can report that her left leg is much closer in size to her right leg. She used to wear thigh-high compression stockings and do work on compression machines every day, but not anymore. And there's no swelling in her legs.

How long should somebody expect that type of change to take? Is it different for each person?

It's different for each person. In the case of my brother, the change occurred in minutes as it was life threatening. For others, change comes within hours, days, or months. In the case of the woman with primary lymphedema, it took years.

Would you share her testimonial with us?

Yes, here it is:

> I was born with primary lymphedema on my left side from the waist down. Secondary symptoms were caused by surgery after an accident.... My parents brought me to Boston's Children's Hospital when I was five to see if anything could be done for me. My left leg was getting bigger and bigger as I grew. While waiting in the hall for the doctors to decide whether or not to cut my leg to make it the same size as the other leg, I believe God sent an angel. A lady passing in the hall saw all of us waiting and said to my parents, "I can see by looking at your little girl why you are here. I have the same condition. Don't let them cut her leg. It will be the worst thing you can do. They did it to me, and the leg just kept growing as I got older."
>
> I'm glad my parents took that leap of faith from what the lady said. It proved to be the right choice. As I grew, my leg kept getting bigger but didn't hinder me until pregnancy weight caused major swelling. And later, as I aged, thigh-high compression stockings became necessary.... My doctor said nothing could be done....
>
> Finally I saw a specialist at Lahey Clinic who suggested massage therapy, which did not help much. I also tried acupuncture with some encouraging results. I initially lost...two inches at the widest measurement on my upper thigh.... Then I started seeing Bhavna in July 2012, and have experienced some amazing results.... As the process began, I asked how she knew what to do. A higher power was instructing her.... Bhavna has helped me to like myself. The people in my life and my family can all see the spiritual and physical changes in me, all for the better.... Bhavna has helped me lose over thirty pounds. I was 154 pounds. I haven't seen this since my wedding forty-five years ago.... Bhavna said no more compression stockings. So I took a leap of faith and got rid of them. To date, my upper left thigh is hovering between nineteen and twenty inches and almost matches my right leg. Our goal is to get the number down to even closer to the right leg, which is now about seven-

teen. I know in my heart, and with the gift that God has given Bhavna to heal people, this will happen.

What a difference you made in her life. It sounds like you kept tuning in to guidance to figure out each step along the way.

Yes. It's hard to explain, but I'm guided by a beautiful power.

Can you describe how you hear or recognize that power? Do you hear a voice or just have a knowing? And how do you have the confidence to follow messages from that power?

Because I've been talking with God for more than sixteen years now. I recognize his voice. I've created a space around me in which I only allow positive energies. When I receive a message to do this or that, I just follow the instructions. It humbles me to be a channel for bringing happiness into people's lives.

Do you ever doubt your abilities or the messages you receive?

Initially, I had some doubts, but now when I'm in the process of healing I just trust it completely and know I am guided to heal people.

When you see positive results repeated over time, then you know you can trust your healing source and process.

Exactly. My treatments have healed almost one thousand people over the years.

When a lot of people hear about energy healing, they don't have a full concept of it. Would you explain more specifically what happens in Reiki?

Reiki is the energy created by what we feel and a universal energy that comes in to help us. We all have both positive and negative parts, or energy, in us. As a Reiki master, I help people connect more to positive energy.

The circumstances, people, and vibrations around us create the way we are and feel. It's our choice how we feel—hurtful or happy, negative or positive. If we choose positive thoughts, we feel happier. If I say to somebody I don't know, "Hey, you're really bad," that person would be taken aback, wonder why I said it, and then be angry or indifferent. The incident would create negative energy around that person. By contrast, telling somebody, "I love you—you're amazing," would create positive energy around them, to which they would immediately respond positively. Even when we are among negative people we can be positive. This reflects a basic principle of life—that every action has an equal and opposite reaction.

I visualize it like sitting in a room with many dots around you—some representing what we view as positive thoughts and others negative thoughts—and getting to choose which ones you're going to tap in to. Having more of what is perceived as negative dots around you makes it harder to focus on the positive dots, but it can be done.

Exactly. What I do as a Reiki master is help people connect to the positive dots. I bring in the exact energy that corresponds with their unique identity. Every person has a unique identity—just like when we receive our Social Security number, which distinguishes us from other people.

When I work on somebody, I move my hands over them with my bracelets jingling. Basically I'm dancing and clearing, and I think the sound and the movement bring in positive energy to shift the vibration to a more positive one.

Is there something people can do for themselves to tune in to the type of energy needed to shift their vibration in this way?

Yes. They can rub the palms of their hands together to produce heat energy. Then slowly move their hands a little apart and feel how the energy is pulling their hands together. They can feel how powerful their energy is by moving their hands apart then closer together.

I feel a tingling sensation and pressure on my palms.

Exactly. The more positive people's thoughts are, the more powerful their energy is. The more negative their thoughts, the less powerful their energy.

An exercise that will immediately center them when stressed at the end of the day and provide more clarity is to bring their hands to their face, hold them there, and take deep breaths. Then, with their eyes closed, bring their hands down to their hearts while again taking deep breaths, and say, "I am good, I am love, and I am peace." I recommend that this be done any time of the day to release stress. It takes less than a minute.

This exercise reminds me of the beauty within me from sitting with myself and touching myself. If we can go into the depth of what's inside of ourselves, then that strength of energy can expand back out and heal anything we're carrying that isn't serving us.

That's right. Too often we get stuck in the smaller part of ourselves. But I believe we all came from one big soul and, when we do this exercise, we're connecting to the bigger part of ourselves and feel that we can deal with anything.

If we were to retest this now by rubbing our hands and separating them, would we feel the sensation on our hands when they are farther apart, as if our aura had expanded?

Yes, every time we do it and the more we do it. I also recommend doing it after drinking water and going to the bathroom, because it relieves stress we're holding in our system.

Like releasing the toxins in our bodies.

Exactly.

What final advice would you like to share about healing that is not commonly thought about?

It's very important to have love for the self. We were all brought up to believe that you're selfish if you do things for yourself. I would say, don't be selfish but learn to love yourself. Then you can selflessly give to others and receive from others.

I agree. If you believe in the principle of unity, you're then loving the piece of that big picture that's yourself.

When you are feeling love in yourself, that's what you're going to project to others, affecting how they will react to you. The more love people have in themselves, the greater its ripple effect will be on the lives of people in the community and the world. Every single person I have met wants to be loved and wants to give love.

I do believe that the motivation behind everything is both to receive and to give love, though sometimes we get a little confused about how to get there.

Right. That's why it's interesting to know that our souls actually come down to give and receive love. When the soul is up there, in the form of a soul, there's no exchange happening, so it comes down and takes the form of a body in order to receive and give love. Different experiences occur in the process, but it is good to let go of them and just connect with the love.

WISDOM TO REMEMBER

If you imagine everything flowing in harmony, it would move like a graceful song and dance just as Bhavna does in her healing work. There is much positive energy in the universe that we can choose to focus on to help us heal from disease, though we all have a unique energy signature and timeline for healing. If you remember learning in science class that all matter is made of energy, you will understand why working at the level of energy can evoke changes as dramatic as those Bhavna has witnessed.

WHAT YOU CAN DO

To reduce stress, become more aware of your positive personal energy, and release toxins after drinking water or going to the bathroom, practice this exercise:

- Rub the palms of your hands together until they feel warm.

- Put your hands over your face.

- Take a few deep breaths.

- While continuing to breathe deeply, close your eyes and bring your hands to your heart.

- Keep breathing deeply and say, "I am good, I am love, and I am peace."

CHAPTER 13

Maintaining Perspective on Medicine

Hyperbaric Oxygen Therapy; Vaccines; and Cures for Cerebral Palsy, Lyme Disease, Brain Injury, and Cervical Cancer

With

K. P. Stoller, MD

"Ethics is nothing else than reverence for life."

—Albert Schweitzer

K. P. Stoller, MD, focuses on functional and integrative medicine. He earned his undergraduate degree from UCLA, where he also did his residency. He specializes in the use of hyperbaric oxygen therapy to treat brain injury—whether from trauma, stroke, autism, cerebral palsy, multiple sclerosis, chemo brain, or Lyme disease. He's a speaker, a faculty member at the Medical Academy of Pediatric Special Needs, and a lifetime fellow of the American College of Hyperbaric Medicine. Interacting with

Dr. Stoller awakened within me the importance of courageously pointing out truths despite the personal risks involved.

Dr. Stoller, what is hyperbaric oxygen therapy?

Hyperbaric oxygen therapy is a therapy done in the chambers that scuba divers use when they get decompression sickness, the bends. Once in the chambers, people are pressurized and usually get 100 percent oxygen.

Would you share a story about someone you helped using hyperbaric oxygen therapy.

My favorite story is about the first little girl I treated with cerebral palsy. She was nine years old, walked like a drunken sailor, and wore braces on her leg. She also had esotropia, a form of strabismus in which one or both eyes turn inward. Cerebral palsy is a static situation neurologically. After about age five, there aren't any spontaneous, miraculous improvements, only a slow grind to attain some neurological and muscular improvements. We treated her with what I call "the brain injury protocol," which is a relatively shallow pressure—seventeen feet below seawater—about as deep as you would want to snorkel if you were in Hawaii. After her first treatment, her eyes aligned. After forty treatments over two months, she had a 40 percent improvement in motor function, a 40 percent improvement in verbal memory, and a 30 percent improvement in visual memory. Her gait normalized, and she got rid of her walking braces. I'm not promising that everyone with cerebral palsy would have such dramatic improvements in just two months, because every brain injury is unique, but that was my experience, over a decade and a half ago, of treating my first patient with cerebral palsy.

Hyperbaric oxygen therapy is not the answer to everything, but that case was about as close to a miracle recovery as you get in such situations. A take-home message might be: "The sooner you can get into a hyperbaric oxygen therapy chamber after neurological injury, the better the recovery is likely to be."

Would you explain more about how hyperbaric oxygen therapy works.

Under pressure, oxygen does things it normally wouldn't do. On a molecular level, it signals the DNA of our cells through oxidative stress. Hyperbaric oxygen therapy is used in hospitals to treat diabetic foot ulcers.

To get new blood vessels and nerves to grow in wounds, you have to signal the DNA. Children with brain injuries, and adults with traumatic brain injuries or who have had strokes, don't actually need to get 100 percent oxygen to signal the DNA. A study done in 2002 in Quebec showed that children with cerebral palsy who were not getting 100 percent oxygen under hyperbaric conditions, but instead compressed room air, improved just as much as children with cerebral palsy who were getting 100 percent oxygen under hyperbaric conditions. There are conditions that do require 100 percent oxygen, but helping repair a brain does not. The portable chambers made out of vinyl are very effective for helping the brain repair itself.

What did the girl with cerebral palsy try before she worked with you?

Physical therapy and occupational therapy.

Was she able to maintain the benefits of the hyperbaric oxygen therapy?

She is doing well, and it's been more than a decade. You don't lose the benefits of the therapy. In fact, I treated a fifteen-year-old boy with fetal alcohol syndrome forty times, and I was doing neurocognitive testing the whole time. I waited for six or seven months before treating him again, then retested him and found he had maintained the gains he made during the first set of treatments. As long as you're not doing something to reinjure or poison the brain, the improvements resulting from the therapy are permanent.

That's great. How can people gain some of the benefits of this technology if they don't have these chambers in their vicinity?

You can rent the chambers. A manufacturer of the portable chambers in California has a rental program. You don't want to drive for hours if you have to be doing this therapy every day anyway, so renting a portable chamber is sometimes the way to go. Now, a portable chamber that only gets up to twelve feet below seawater pressure is not the right depth to treat gas gangrene or a diabetic foot ulcer, but that pressure's okay for treating a stroke, or a traumatic brain injury, or cerebral palsy.

What else might a person do to help with brain injury?

Many nutritional things can help, such as various supplements, omega-3s, and curcumin, the active ingredient in turmeric. Even if you're just taking the curcumin or turmeric in capsule form, it's always best to take it with hot food or hot tea, because that will bring out the Ayurvedic medicinal qualities of the spice. There are other ways to help the brain recover as well, but nothing as dramatic as hyperbaric oxygen therapy.

What is the best form of omega-3 to take?

A fish oil supplement is best unless you're a vegetarian, in which case you can get omega-3s from algae. There are companies that sell algae-based DHAs, but they are not as concentrated as the ones from fish oil.

You mention on your website that politics and science are inseparable. What does that mean in terms of medicine and healing?

Politics has become wedded to science; science has been taken over by corporations. We're basically living in an age of false prophets, where you cannot believe what authorities are telling you.

How can people determine which resources are trustworthy? One way is to check who funded and conducted the research, right?

Right, but sometimes researchers do not reveal conflicts of interest. For example, Dr. Paul Offit, of Children's Hospital in Philadelphia, often doesn't disclose when he goes on various talk shows or writes columns that he's a patent holder of vaccines from which he has profited, and is appointed to an endowed chair from a pharmaceutical company. He's basically being paid to be a mouthpiece for pharmaceutical interests, yet he's portrayed as a professor of infectious diseases at Children's Hospital. Mainstream media is not the place to go for the truth anymore.

Let's focus on information about some specific conditions. What is the root cause of Lyme disease, and what does it lead to?

Lyme disease is actually a pandemic plague that is occurring now, and part of what makes it a plague in the biblical sense is the global negation of this illness. Probably more than 18 percent of the world's population is infected with *Borrelia* which is a *genus* of bacteria of the spirochete phylum. It causes *Borreliosis*, a zoonotic, vector-borne disease transmitted primarily by ticks. If you were to say to people, "Hey, you have to have one of these two diseases—do you want syphilis or do you want Lyme?" people will pick Lyme, because they don't know anything about it. But Lyme disease is syphilis on steroids. You can get rid of syphilis with a shot of penicillin. Lyme disease does not go away easily, and it's very difficult to detect and much more insidious than syphilis. It doesn't give you some ugly lesion on your genitalia, but it can cause arthritis, chronic fatigue, muscle wasting, neuropathies, as well as get in your brain and make you bipolar, psychotic or give you ADD.

Some physicians, even at prestigious universities, don't believe it's an illness, but the Centers for Disease Control (CDC) will tell you that 330,000 new cases of Lyme disease occur every year. This figure suggests that we're dealing with maybe 50 million Americans who have this illness, most of whom are asymptomatic, just as 90 percent of people with tuberculosis are asymptomatic. But eventually your immune system has a bad day, and once the Lyme organism gets hold of a person it doesn't let go.

There are two problems in getting rid of Lyme disease. First, it slathers itself with biofilm, like the stuff you brush off your teeth every day, and even the right antibiotics have trouble penetrating biofilm. Second, this organism leaves persister cells. They can become inert, and you can't kill it because it doesn't have any metabolic activity. It has one eye open, waiting for the coast to be clear, then it restarts the infection. There's no test for persister cells, so you don't know if you have them. You just have to be vigilant about symptoms coming back after you've successfully treated the illness, whether it's two weeks, two months, or twenty years later.

What is the treatment for Lyme disease?

There are lots of treatments, but some are better than others. If ever there was a time to be aggressive and use antibiotics, it is with Lyme disease, but this is problematic for people whose constitutions can't take multiple antibiotics at one time. Hyperbaric oxygen therapy kills the organism. You could actually use hyperbaric oxygen therapy as an antibiotic, but when you have Lyme disease often you don't just have Borreliosis but also other infections. Also, hyperbaric oxygen doesn't address co-infections such as Babesia, transmitted by a parasitic protozoan, or Bartonella, "cat scratch fever," both co-infections that can go along with Lyme disease.

People are also faced with the dilemma of getting diagnosed correctly. For example, in the San Francisco Bay Area half the infected ticks have *Borrelia miyamotoi*, which will cause Lyme disease but not test positive on the conventional test for Lyme disease. The conventional test for Lyme disease, the ELISA test, can miss up to 60 percent of infected patients, while the Western blot can miss up to 90 percent. If you have *Borrelia miyamotoi*, which is not a *Borrelia burgdorferi* group organism (classic Lyme disease) but a relapsing fever *Borrelia genus*, it will be missed by the Lyme disease test yet clinically you could be even sicker than someone with *Borrelia burgdorferi*.

I'm sure there are hundreds and hundreds, or thousands, of people out there who have been told they don't have Lyme and actually do. If you don't go to a Lyme-literate doctor, you're likely not going to be diagnosed correctly. Most people who get bitten by ticks don't even know it because they're getting bitten by little nymphs that are no larger than a pinhead, although when they get bitten by an adult tick they usually know about it. And ticks are not the only way to get Lyme disease. It can be transmitted congenitally, so a mother can pass it on to her infant. Technically, it can also be transmitted through sexual contact, but it's not transmitted as much sexually as syphilis is. If you have relations with Sally Syphilis, I think you're going to get syphilis every time, but Linda Lyme probably will not give you Lyme disease even half the time. We don't know if the odds of this happening are 1 in 500, 1 in 5,000, or 1 in half a million. But it is definitely possible.

Is there a direct test for *Borrelia miyamotoi*?

There's a direct test and an indirect test. A direct test means you're looking for the organism's DNA. The recognized test for Lyme disease is indirect, which means you're looking at antibody levels. I don't usually use a direct test because there's a 70 percent chance of that test giving a false negative. The Lyme organism does not like to hang out in your blood. It likes to go to oxygen-deprived areas of the body, such as joints, synovial fluid, muscles, bone marrow, or sinuses. If you line up ten people who you know have Lyme disease and you look for the DNA of the organism in their blood, you'll have only a 30 percent chance of finding it. It's not a test we can use as an outcome measure. You could take the test today, find out you have Lyme disease, do nothing, repeat the test in two weeks, and be negative. If at that point you think you don't have Lyme disease anymore, you'll be wrong.

This is really a serious infectious disease problem, and the CDC hasn't done anything significant about it for thirty years except watch it get worse. But telling the American people the truth about the Lyme disease situation today is problematic for the CDC. Let's say you were an ethical member of the Infectious Disease Division of the CDC and wanted to tell the American people the real story. Are you going to make an announcement, saying the following? "We wanted to let you know that probably as many as fifty million Americans are infected with a bacterium that can kill you, give you all kinds of mental illnesses, Alzheimer's disease, and oh, we don't really have a good test to diagnose it or a consensus on treatment for it. Have a nice evening." A message like that is going to cause people to lose sleep.

It's not that the CDC doesn't mind scaring people, but there's no pharmaceutical company in a position to make big bucks by having the CDC announce the truth about Lyme disease. Most of the drugs used to treat it are generic. In fact, the government would stand to lose a lot of money if the truth were known because it would be more difficult to deny disability claims and 3rd party payers would have a harder time refusing to reimburse for treatment.

Hyperbaric oxygen therapy is an alternative treatment for Lyme disease. There are also a lot of herbs that can help, but I wouldn't count on herbs eradicating the infection. In addition, diet is important to assist detoxification. Anything that improves the immune system will help.

What are some herbs that can help?

There's Teasel root, Samento root, cat's claw, Banderol and garlic. Various companies sell herbs and other forms of relief for people with Lyme disease. A lot of these alternative therapies make people feel better, such as the salt and vitamin C therapy, which will clear out a lot of parasites and reset any dysbiosis you might be having in your gut. Since the gut is 70 percent of your immune system, it helps your immune system, but it's not going to get the Lyme organism out of your bone marrow. Good results can come from a lot of these therapies, but you still need the big guns.

For some people, if they're not careful the cure is worse than the disease, because they can get a severe reaction when their immune system goes topsy-turvy as the antibiotics start killing the organisms. The first third of my book *Incurable Me* is devoted to Lyme disease because it's so pervasive.

Have you seen the movie *Under Our Skin* and its sequel, which are about Lyme disease?

I've seen part one several times. My favorite scene that I tell patients about is where a park ranger says about his Lyme disease treatment, "Finally, after two years, my antibiotics kicked in." It took two years for the antibiotics to work because of the biofilm of the Lyme organism. My favorite drug is Alinia, which is licensed by the FDA to treat certain protozoal parasites, such as Giardia. Babesia is a protozoa and one of the Lyme co-infections. Alinia does a good job of destroying biofilm on several different types of bacteria, including the Lyme disease organism. But only about 30 percent of people can use Alinia by itself to get rid of their Borreliosis.

What aspects of diet help treat Lyme disease?

You don't want to eat anything that has a deleterious effect on your immune system, so you don't want to drink alcohol or consume foods with refined sugar. Because pesticides are another big problem, you want to eat organic foods. When I was writing my book, I asked the question: "Why would one person get Alzheimer's disease from Lyme disease and another not?" It's because of neurospirochetes—90 to 100 percent of autopsied brains from Alzheimer's disease patients have a neurospirochetosis, and 25 percent of those organisms have been identified as the Lyme disease–causing organism *Borrelia burgdorferi*. Recently, Kris Kristofferson announced that the Alzheimer's disease he thought he had two years ago was actually Lyme disease. There are spirochetes in the mouth, and they're benign; but if you get Lyme disease these organisms have strands of DNA called plasmids. The Lyme organism can shoot out and share these plasmids, as if they were on the Internet, with other members of its genus and other spirochetes, causing these otherwise benign oral spirochetes to become more virulent and get into your brain. Regarding this problem, conventional medicine is completely asleep at the wheel.

The CDC says there are three hundred thirty thousand new cases of Lyme disease every year, so why don't we have a vaccine for Lyme disease? People have been getting money for trying to make one for the past twenty years, but for a vaccine to fit an illness model, the vaccine induced antibodies has to help eradicate the organism—if antibodies alone can't get rid of the infection what good is the vaccine. There is more to the immune system than antibodies and often vaccines don't even do a good job at stimulating antibodies.

Could you share a little more about the positive and negative effects of vaccines that we are told we and our children need.

First and foremost, the vaccine programs are a multibillion-dollar windfall to pharmaceutical companies, and if they can get a vaccine mandated by the CDC they have no liability for any untoward reactions to it. There are two or three hundred vaccines in the pipeline for just about everything, because this is a cash cow. There are even accusations that vaccines are being used for biological warfare. For example, there are reports that in the Philippines, Nigeria, and Kenya, the World Health Organization has put human chorionic gonadotropin into tetanus vaccines given to childbearing-age women as a population-control agent, sterilizing them without their permission.

Some people feel that the risk of vaccines having a damaging effect on the body might be greater than the risk of getting the diseases the vaccines are supposed to protect us from.

Yes. For example, let's look at the meningitis vaccine that a lot of colleges want their students to get. While you can die from getting Neisseria meningitis, if you look at the CDC's projection of who's going to have side effects and how many untoward deaths might occur from this vaccine, you find that for every potential case of meningitis you're preventing, two people will die and one thousand children will have severe adverse events. So, it's better for people to take their chances of getting meningitis than imposing the vaccine on the population. You don't mandate an intervention that will double the number of potential deaths and cause one thousand severe adverse events for one case that is being prevented.

What about some of the other vaccines?

There is the HPV vaccine. The package insert the vaccine clinic receives says 40 girls died in clinical trials out of 29,000 subjects. That is actually 64 times the death rate of dying from cervical cancer in the USA. And there is no proof the vaccine actually prevents cervical cancer. However, cervical cancer is a nutritional disease, and if people have adequate vitamin D levels they are not likely to get cervical cancer. But you don't see anybody passing out vitamin D to women, because that's not going to make anybody rich. If you do get cervical dysplasia, there are things you can take from nature, such as Indole-3-carbinol, found in cruciferous vegetables like broccoli, Brussels sprouts, and cabbage. If you eat one-third of a head of cabbage every day, you get about 400 milligrams of Indole-3-carbinol, which gives you a chance of reversing cervical dysplasia.

There's also been a fairly benign drug called isoprinosine available for decades everywhere but in the United States. This drug has been shown to eliminate cancer-causing strains of HPV within two weeks. The HPV vaccine was never needed; the alternatives have always been better. The vaccine actually increases your chances of getting cancer from the strains that the vaccine doesn't protect against.

We should never lose the ability to have informed consent, but certain factions of the CDC and the government want to be able to vaccinate us with whatever whenever they want. It's not like those vaccines are benign and one size fits all. That is a violation of human rights even if the vaccines performed as advertised, but they often do not. The flu vaccine has a 10% efficacy rating. That means it doesn't work 90% of the time. Hospitals are firing staff because they won't get a vaccine that has a 90% failure rating.

What can we do on our own to keep ourselves healthy?

We can vote with our dollars regarding the foods we buy, refusing to buy foods that are not organic or that have been sprayed with glyphosate. If we can't eat organic grains, we should not eat them. We can find out what's in our food and stop trusting corporations to control the seed and pesticides. Giving other people such power over our diets can cost us our health.

Today, there are many ways to farm at home, even growing just a few plants indoors, so that we know our vegetables and fruits are fresh and organic. Also, growing some of our own food at home creates a mindset focused on our health and well-being, certainly a beneficial attitude.

WISDOM TO REMEMBER

Dr. K. P. Stoller shines a spotlight on the importance of understanding the political and economic aspects of medicine and how they can impact our choices for healing.

While taking drugs puts unnatural substances in your body, often just treats symptoms rather than the underlying cause of a disease, and has side effects, there are times when those side effects may pose less risk than the disease itself, such as taking antibiotics for Lyme disease.

When vaccines are made mandatory, the principle of informed consent is negated. People can remember their right to decline vaccines that have done more harm than good.

WHAT YOU CAN DO

Hyperbaric oxygen therapy is helpful for healing cerebral palsy, brain injury, and Lyme disease. If you cannot find a medical facility with a hyperbaric oxygen chamber, you can buy or rent a portable one. You can also aid the healing process with food, supplements, and herbs, which, although unlikely to eradicate the problem on their own, can reduce symptoms and strengthen the body.

Here are some suggestions to discuss with your doctor and see if they are right for you.

- To help detect Lyme disease Dr. Stoller is exclusively referring his patients to IgeneX Lab's Immunoblot testing procedure. A separate test that can be ordered as well is the antibody test to help detect *Borrelia* in the Relapsing Fever group.

- To help heal Lyme disease, try a combination of the following:

  ~ Antibiotics

  ~ Hyperbaric oxygen therapy

- ~ Alinia, licensed by the FDA to treat protozoa like *Babesia,* since it breaks through the biofilm blocking antibiotics from getting at the Lyme organism

- ~ No refined sugar

- ~ Organic foods

- ~ Thistle root

- ~ Cat's claw

- To help heal brain injury in general, try:

  - ~ Omega-3 supplements—fish oil for nonvegetarians; algae for vegetarians

  - ~ Curcumin, or turmeric, taken with hot food or hot tea

- To help prevent cervical cancer:

  - ~ Maintain an adequate level of vitamin D in your body

  - ~ Use Isoprinosine, which has shown to eliminate cancer-causing strains of HPV within two weeks

- To help treat cervical dysplasia:

  - ~ Take Indole-3-carbinol

  - ~ Eat broccoli, Brussels sprouts, and cabbage

PART V

Emotions, Spirituality, and Healing

CHAPTER 14

Reason to Live

SELF-INDUCED HEALING OF CANCER

With

BERNIE SIEGEL, MD

"My religion is very simple. My religion is kindness."

—Dalai Lama

Bernie Siegel, MD, has transitioned from being a pediatric surgeon to running support groups and being a life coach. He has written numerous books, including *Love, Medicine and Miracles*. He developed a therapy program called Exceptional Cancer Patients, in which he utilizes patients' drawings, dreams, images, and feelings to create a system of care-frontation. He has been designated one of the top twenty spiritually influential people by *Watkins Review*.

Am I right, you prefer being called Bernie?

I feel that my relationship with patients should be on an equal footing. It doesn't seem right that I call patients by their first names and they have to say Dr. Siegel, as if MD stands for "medical deity."

How do you go about helping people heal beyond what typically happens in a doctor's office?

I went into medicine because I care about people, but then it was painful because I couldn't cure everything. So I sought other ways of helping patients, such as establishing a group to teach what I now call "survival behavior." I sent one hundred letters to people with cancer, saying, "You want to live a longer, better life, come to a meeting." This wasn't promising them anything beyond sharing things I had learned. Only twelve women came to the first meeting. That's when I realized I don't know the people I'm taking care of. They're afraid of failing, thinking, *What if I go to his group and don't get well?* Psychiatrists know their patients better than oncologists because they care for people from an emotional and lifestyle perspective.

I often recall the words of a lawyer who once said, "While learning to think, I almost forgot how to feel." This lawyer, who had cancer, said he had a 5 percent chance of living two years. In a bookstore, my book fell off the shelf into his hand and transformed his life. His cancer disappeared. He said to his doctor, "Do you want to know what I did?" The doctor said, "No." That, to me, is tragic. Doctors call such transformations spontaneous remissions. But it wasn't spontaneous. In his book *Cancer Ward*, Russian novelist Aleksandr Solzhenitsyn used a wonderful term that woke me up—"self-induced healing."

Like that lawyer, people can transform their lives by creating rhythm and harmony instead of stress, sending a different message to their bodies. A lot of damage comes from emotional turmoil, which depletes your immune system and all your body chemistry. When there is an emotional drain, rest doesn't replace it. Why are adults having more heart attacks, suicides, and strokes on Monday? Kids knock themselves out, but they're loving what they're doing, so they're not coming down with illness.

Doctors tend to treat patients like physical things. When repairing cars, mechanics work on parts of them. We call electricians or plumbers to fix specific problems in houses. But we are not cars or houses. We're mind and body units, and doctors need to treat the units rather than expecting a psychiatrist to address a mental problem while we address a physical problem.

If you have depression following a family tragedy, the doctor gives you an antidepressant without even asking why you're depressed. Turning depression into something mechanical by simply treating physical symptoms doesn't benefit people, while helping them heal their lives does provide physical benefits.

Would you tell us about somebody you helped heal beyond what we normally see in the practice of medicine.

One of my first lessons was years ago with a landscaper, John, who was retiring and had developed an ulcer. Doctors assumed it had been caused by stress because he was about to make a big transition in his life.

John's ulcer didn't heal, so the doctors did an endoscopy and biopsy, and discovered it was cancer, not just a stress ulcer. I said, "John, you've been walking around with this thing for quite a while. We've got to get you in the hospital and get it out of there." He replied, "You forgot something." I asked, "What did I forget?" He responded, "It's springtime. I'm going home to make the world beautiful, so if I die I'll leave a beautiful world." He wasn't trying not to die but was focused on making the world beautiful.

A few weeks later he came back and said, "Okay, I'm ready." After the surgery and the report, I had to tell him, "I couldn't get all the cancer out. You need to get chemotherapy, maybe radiation." He replied, "No, you forgot something." I asked, "What did I forget this time?" He responded: "It's still springtime. I don't have time for more treatments. I'm going home to make the world beautiful. If I die, I'll leave a beautiful world." And he left.

One day six years later the nurse in our office handed me John's chart. I said, "He must be dead; he never came back. We must have two patients with the same name. Get the other chart." She replied, "Bernie, open the door." So I opened the door, and there sat John, who said, "I have a hernia from lifting boulders in my landscape business." I took care of his hernia.

Then John became my teacher. I spent a lot of time with him, walking in the woods and seeing how beautiful the world was through his eyes. He changed me; after that, while jogging or biking I would pull up little plants because they looked so pretty I wanted to put them in my yard. John lived well into his nineties. When his wife died, he turned off his switch, so to speak, and died shortly thereafter. I spoke at their seventieth wedding anniversary, telling people how John had taught me to appreciate the beauty in the world. Seeing beauty and valuing relationships are common themes in the lives of people who enjoy health and longevity.

By contrast, once a husband, wife, and two children were in the office, and the husband had cancer. He said, "There's no point in living. I can't work anymore." I replied, "Look to your left. There are three good reasons." As if I had hit him in the head with a mallet, he suddenly appreciated his family.

Another cancer patient, a woman, had twelve cats. Her kids told me: "The house smells, and it's a mess. We got to get rid of the cats. She'll be on chemotherapy, and we've got to protect her." I said, "No, what you need to do is keep the house clean. If you take those cats away, your mother will die. But if you say to her, 'Nobody wants twelve cats,' she can't die." They saw that what I was saying was true and, during another visit, remarked, "You were right. It was a good thing we cleaned up yet left her the cats."

Then there was a lady who said, "I have nine kids. I can't die until they're all married and out of the house." Her cancer came back twenty years later when her last child had left home. When she didn't have the role of mother anymore, her body chemistry changed. It's as if when there's no reason to live, your body determines it will end your life.

Survival is often about attitudes and beliefs, whether it's going to Lourdes or some healer halfway around the world or traveling to be in a beautiful location. One man said to me, "I'm going to go to Colorado to die in the mountains because it's beautiful there." A year later I called his family to ask why I hadn't been invited to the funeral, and he answered, "It's so beautiful here I forgot to die."

Another man bought a house on the beach in Florida just to have a beautiful place to meditate during the last few months of his life. He lived for over five years and became a teacher at his hospital.

I have a letter from a patient who wrote, "I bought a dog and put in a backyard wildlife habitat, laughed more, took vitamins, didn't die, and now I'm so busy I'm killing myself." It's important to follow your heart—regarding treatment or anything else.

I've had patients who accepted God as their resource and stopped worrying and fearing, such as a woman with a large tumor who said, "I'm going home to die." Then one day many months later, she came to the office and reported that she had gone home and left her troubles to God and her tumor had disappeared.

One of my teachers said that the people most likely to survive cancer are single moms and the next most likely are moms.

Absolutely. Also, loving and being loved affects health, and that includes loving yourself. What I say to the moms is, "Don't just be a mom, be your own kid." In other words, care for yourself too, so that you have your own life. Harvard students participating in a study were asked, "Did your parents love you?" Ninety-eight percent of those who said no suffered a major illness by middle age. Only twenty-four percent of those who answered yes suffered a major illness.

One time a woman wearing a bright iridescent red outfit that was giving me a headache was sitting in the front row while I was lecturing. I wondered why she had worn such an outfit. Then she handed me a letter, and when I read it I understood. It said:

> My mother told me I was a failure, that I'd never amount to anything. She dressed me in dark clothes so nobody would ever notice me. My mother's words were eating away at me and maybe gave me cancer. When I developed cancer, I started reading your books, and you gave me the permission to become my authentic self. So I went out and bought a red dress and some red high-heeled shoes.

I forgave her for what she was wearing and said to her, "You didn't need my permission." Now whenever I lecture near where she lives, I know she'll show up at the event wearing a red outfit, and I'll ask her to stand up and tell her story.

I was fortunate to have grown up with loving parents and grandparents. As a result, I initially didn't realize the difficulties other people go through growing up. In one study, 70 percent of high school students said that they had contemplated suicide. One lawyer told me that he wanted to be a violinist but his parents had said, "No, we can't be proud of a violinist. We want you to go to law school." So he became a lawyer and eventually got cancer. Then he got a job at an orchestra and didn't die when he was supposed to. People need to claim their own lives. I tell patients, "Don't lose your life to make other people happy."

How do you recommend people interact with loved ones who have cancer so that they maintain the hope necessary for healing?

I can tell you what I've learned while dealing with two family members. First, many decades ago my wife developed multiple sclerosis (MS). A neurologist met me in the hospital cafeteria and told me what was going to happen to my wife. I thought, *Why aren't we in the doctor's office so I can display emotion, cry?* Then I realized he couldn't handle an emotional situation so he wanted to tell me in front of people in the hospital cafeteria, where we couldn't react emotionally. Of course, what he had predicted didn't happen.

Many years later one of our children, at age seven, said, "I need an X-ray." I asked, "What are you talking about?" He said, "My knee hurts." I replied, "I've been telling you, take a hot bath and it'll feel better." But he kept insisting he needed an X-ray.

As it turned out, he was listening to his intuition, or inner wisdom. We got an X-ray, which showed he had a bone tumor that looked malignant. I thought, *They'll be cutting his leg off and then he'll probably die in a year or two because I've been telling him to take a bath instead of treating the leg.* I was feeling guilty and sad thinking we were going to lose a child.

The day after I told my family about the X-ray, our son said to me, "Dad, can I talk to you for a minute?" I replied, "Sure, what is it?" He responded, "You're handling this poorly. Look, we're trying to have a nice day and play in the front yard, and you want us in our bedroom worrying about next year. We're not going to worry about next year." He taught me a lot. And as it turned out, my son's tumor was benign and he was fine.

Then eight years later an abnormal mammogram revealed that my wife had cancer. I thought, *I'm not going to worry about what will happen next year, five years from now.* I stopped some of the treatments she was put on, because her MS was making her feel even more tired. "How can you do that?" some of her doctors asked me. I replied, "Don't you know that what you're giving her is no good? She's on hormones and other things to keep her as young and healthy as possible." Experiences like this have reoriented me to care for individuals, not treat diseases. We need to continually emphasize that patients are human beings and have complex life histories.

Doctors sometimes forget they're treating people. At times in the hospital doctors will say, "How's room 422?" I'll reply, "What are you talking about? The room is in good condition. What about the person?"

I often say to patients, "Bring your baby pictures and put them up around the room so doctors see you as a person, not just a patient." Rarely do these patients end up dying due to a medical error, which is one of the leading causes of death in the United States.

Attitudes and beliefs can truly affect outcomes. One doctor using a chemotherapy agent that began with the letters EPO and ended with H, called the "EPOH protocol," realized that by turning the letters around it spelled *hope*. So he started calling his treatment the "hope protocol." As a result, three or four times as many patients responded positively to the treatment.

Once, an upset doctor told me that he repaired the radiation therapy machine but forgot to put the radioactive material back in, and gave patients treatments anyway before noticing his error. Yet patients' tumors were shrinking, and the patients had the usual side effects of the treatments they thought they were getting. It's about the beliefs.

I always encourage people to draw pictures about their diseases and treatments to show their inner feelings about them. Patients who draw an X-ray machine as a devil giving them poison usually experience every side effect in the book. But those who draw treatments coming from God tend to have no side effects. A lot of these people have been called "Siegel's crazy patients," which I regard as a complimentary term showing that other doctors realized the power of the beliefs held by these patients and why they were doing so much better than other patients.

How does the drawing therapy work?

I started encouraging patients to do drawings to reveal their inner feelings and awaken self-awareness. When I was burying my feelings as a doctor, Elisabeth Kübler-Ross, the renowned Swiss-American psychiatrist, asked me to draw an outdoor scene. Her first question was, "Why is eleven important?" I said, "Why do you ask?" She replied, "Well, there are eleven trees in the picture." Numbers are a way we store memories. Jung said numbers have meaning—that, for example, a person has a traumatic event at a certain age and that number can show up in a drawing. Then she asked, "What are you covering up?" I said, "What are you talking about?" She replied, "I gave you a white piece of paper, and you used a white crayon to make snow on the mountain. You added a layer, so what are you covering up?" I was hiding my feelings. Because of what Elisabeth taught me about drawings, I now realize that color and numbers have meaning and the quadrants on the page relate to time. Drawings often awaken self-awareness in patients. For example, if a patient says to me, "I'm going to take this job in Wisconsin" or "I'm going to marry her and move to Vermont" or "I'm going to have chemotherapy," I might say, "Draw yourself in that situation." And if the drawing looks horrible—depicting the person in a prison or black room, for example—I might say, "This may not be a good choice for you."

If the patient says, "I want to go ahead," I might say, "All right, then, three or four times a day picture yourself going forward and everything turning out beautifully." Then a week or two later I might ask the person to make another drawing of the situation, and it would be beautiful because they had been reprogrammed. At this point I'll say, "Intuitively, you know it's the right thing for you." When people are living in fear of a particular course of action yet suddenly aware of knowing it's the right thing to do, they can reprogram themselves, after which everything will turn out all right.

Drawings can even help me know when people are going to die—perhaps indicated by a purple kite or balloon going up in the sky. (Purple is a spiritual color, yet drawing in purple doesn't mean the person is dying.) Once a four-year-old named Amber, who had been through many treatments in an attempt to save her life, made a drawing of a purple balloon with colorful dots all around it going up out of the picture. A few weeks later I got a call from her mother, who said Amber had told her, "I'm dying today as a gift to you, to free you from all the trouble." That day was her mother's birthday, and the number of colorful dots exactly matched the days that had been left in her life.

A nurse also drew a picture with a purple kite going up in the sky and four pretty trees. Her husband was flying the kite, so I had him come in and said, "Your wife is ready to go, but see, you're hanging on to the kite." He replied, "Yeah, my wife's a nurse and she takes care of everything. I don't know how to make a meal, pay the bills, or do anything around the house. So she said, "I won't die; I'll train you." Four months later he came to her and said, "Honey, I cut the string, and if you need to go it's okay." She replied, "Then I'll die Thursday, when the kids get here from California," and so she did.

A child who had cancer said, "My family doesn't give me any time." I said, "Draw a picture of your family." She drew herself in a purple outfit sitting on a chair all alone. The rest of the family was on the sofa with an empty seat, where she could have been. Their arms were around the other kids or folded up. I showed it to the parents, and they were so grateful to know what their child was feeling. Years later they called me and said, "We want to thank you. Before she died, we spent a lot of time with her, and it was wonderful to be able to do that rather than have her die feeling like we didn't love her."

It's important that doctors take the time to observe and call attention to aspects of patients' lives that could be improved to create better conditions for healing. One day in my office a young suicidal woman said, "You're my CD." I asked, "What do you mean?" She replied, "You're my chosen dad." So now I say to people who might benefit from such support, "I'll be your CD. I'll be your chosen dad."

It doesn't mean I like what patients are doing if they're not taking care of themselves, but I will still love them. I have seen this tactic turn some patients around, especially those who have experienced the opposite of love—such as indifference, rejection, or abuse.

I also say to patients, "I'll see you next week" or "I'll see you in two weeks." It may take months to sink in, but eventually they think, *This guy cares about me, so maybe I'm worth something.* Then they start taking care of themselves. And when they act self-destructive, I laugh and say, "It's obvious you're trying to get my attention," so they know that I noticed what they were doing.

Once when I was a police surgeon in New Haven, a police officer called and said, "Doctor Siegel, I'm going to commit suicide." What popped out of my mouth was, "If you commit suicide, I'll never speak to you again," and I hung up the phone, figuring there was nothing I could do. A sermon was not going to work with him. About fifteen minutes later the policeman, who had been a professional football player, came crashing into my office screaming so much about how insensitive I'd been that I thought he was going to throw me out the window. I said, "Do you realize you're not dead?" Immediately he understood that my initial comment had been said on purpose, indicating that it had worked.

I also have remarks from another suicidal patient recorded on my answering machine, saying: "Do you have Jack Kevorkian's phone number? My father's abused me sexually. I have a brain tumor. I want to be dead." I called her back and told her, "I love you. You'll be my chosen daughter." She's alive today and sent me a card with the following message: "A smile ran across my face today because you ran across my mind…. I think of you every day—you're an angel in my life. All my love." It's a wonderful feeling to know that you've helped someone feel better because they feel love.

I also advise people to become love warriors, telling people who are in conflict with them, "I love you." I always say, "Even if somebody's screaming at you for taking their parking space, lower your window and say, "I love you." That will get them to leave. One woman, who had alcoholic parents, cancer, and a life of abuse, started saying "I love you" to her parents but they wouldn't answer her. Then one day she came in and said, "I was late for work today, so I ran out of the house, and my parents were in the street screaming, 'You forgot something. You didn't say I love you today.' We were hugging and crying in the street."

Once when Mother Teresa was invited to an antiwar rally, she said, "I won't attend. But if you ever have a peace rally call me." She was saying the same thing I'm saying: Don't fight a war against disease; instead, heal your life and your body. It's a totally different perspective.

WISDOM TO REMEMBER

Bernie Siegel, MD, brings us back to our humanity by emphasizing that patients are people—mind and body units—not physical objects or room numbers, and that treating your emotional issues can heal your physical issues. He also stresses the impact of attitudes and beliefs on healing, reminding us that instead of fighting disease it is more helpful to focus on what brings beauty, harmony, and peace to our lives.

Three key contributors to healing and longevity are:

- Having a reason to live

- Loving your life, yourself, and giving to and receiving love from others

- Believing that treatments will heal you

WHAT YOU CAN DO

- Do what you love with the same amount of joy a child would.

- Follow the treatment plan you truly believe will help you heal.

- Say "I love you" to people with whom you may be in conflict.

- When in the hospital, put your baby photos on the wall so doctors remember you as a person.

- Draw pictures to better understand how you feel about situations in your life and treatment prospects. The colors you select, numbers of items you depict, and the placement of people and objects all may have symbolic meaning, offering increased insight into your past, present, and future circumstances.

CHAPTER 15

The Mandala—Window to Your Soul

CANCER DOES NOT EQUAL DEATH

With

MAMIE-JEAN LAMLEY

"As I say yes to life, life says yes to me."

—Louise Hay

Mamie-Jean Lamley, a powerful businesswoman, runs the training business Empowerment on Fire, as well as the spiritual business Mandala Mystics: The Window to Your Soul. She also works at events hosted by Success Resources, a leading global transformation and education company. When I see her at work, she maintains an inner sense of calm with a big smile and powerful focused action. Her use of mandalas in her own healing from cancer and in helping others face the challenges of illness is remarkable.

Mamie, would you tell us about your journey of healing.

The disease from which I recovered—and am now thriving as a result of working with mandalas—is cervical cancer. I grew up in Hawaii and have had many aunts and uncles die of various forms of cancer, so when my doctor told me at age thirty-five that I had cervical cancer, the world seemed to come to a stop. In most people's minds, cancer equals death, and that was not what I wanted to happen! I finally had three beautiful children I had waited for ever since doctors had told me I couldn't have children. All I had to say was, "I can't die. I have three beautiful children, and we have a whole lifetime ahead of us."

Why did the doctors tell you that you could not have children?

My pelvis was tilted a certain way, so they believed that I would not be able to have children. It was heartbreaking for me because I loved children. But I just said to myself, "One day I *will* have children." Meanwhile, I took care of everybody else's children. When one door closes, you have to find another way to realize your dreams and get what you want out of life. So instead of being sad, I devoted time to my nieces and nephews.

Then at age twenty-seven I was blessed with the birth of my first child. She weighed eleven pounds, which fixed the problem the doctors thought was preventing me from having children! So by the time I was thirty-five I was blessed with three children.

It seems like that was your first miracle.

When someone tells us that we can't do something, it's amazing how we say, "Well, just watch me." That's what I did.

When I got word that I had cervical cancer, they told me it was stage 2, then during my first exam they said, "We think it's stage three or four." When some people hear they're in stage 3 or stage 4, they give up, but I was raised to show determination and to go beyond expectations.

The day I was told that I had cancer I was actually on stage teaching a course called Think Like a Leader and doing what I love: training people. My assistant took the call from my doctor, who mentioned cancer and told her, "We need to talk to Mamie right away." My assistant asked me if I could have the class go on break because I needed to take the call. So I announced a fifteen-minute break and took the call. The doctor said, "Mamie, we need you to come to the hospital as soon as possible because we believe you have a progressive case of cervical cancer." With my heart racing, I told him, "I have to finish my class first. I will be there at about five-thirty."

I didn't have time to digest the news because my students were coming back from the break, so I told them I needed a ten-minute personal break and went to the bathroom. There I broke down and said to myself, "Cancer does not equal death. There's a reason for this." After a good cry, I took my makeup out of my bag and put my face back on, then went to finish my four-hour class. Because my students were wondering what was going on, I told them at the end of class, "I just want you to know that this has been a great day. Now I need to go to the hospital since the doctors believe I have a form of cancer. But I'll deal with it." They embraced me with so much love and support it was unbelievable.

I can feel it as if you're speaking to them right now.

I called my mom and told her I was heading to the hospital. She was in a panic, thinking that her child should never pass before she did. I told her, "Mom, I'm not passing! But I'd love to have you on my side. Can you meet me at the hospital?" There I was, thirty-five years old and asking my mom to help me.

One of the lessons I learned was when you are diagnosed with an illness that could be terminal you need to surround yourself with the people who make a difference in your life. Having my mom by my side as I went through the initial diagnosis and all the tests that came after, put me in the space of: this is temporary—we will get through it.

Once I knew exactly what I had, I did my own research. I then asked my medical doctors if I could work with my naturopathic doctor. I wanted both worlds to come together for the sake of my health and wellness.

On the medical side, they were recommending surgery, hoping to go in, freeze the cancer cells, and cut them out. The test results following that surgery made me think they got everything. But when further test results came back three days later, they told me the cancer wasn't all gone and they needed to take out everything. That was the hardest part. I thought, *Every doctor told me I couldn't have children, but I have three children. I'm good. If they need to take everything else out, so be it.*

They removed my uterus and one ovary, leaving the other ovary so that I could produce estrogen. But they said within five years that ovary would have to come out, too. The scariest part was that they weren't sure if the cancer cells had spread to other organs.

All the while, I was in Hawaii and that meant my kids, who were in Colorado, would be without a mother for six months. At first they had the same mindset that I'd had: cancer equals death. It was hard knowing they thought they were going to lose their mother.

Before my second surgery, upon hearing the doctors say they didn't get everything after all, I felt like I was having a mental breakdown. That's when I turned inward to gain inner peace, realizing that if I wasn't calm I couldn't expect those supporting me to be calm.

Following my third surgery, the doctors confirmed that no cancer cells were found on any other internal organs and I would go through oral chemotherapy. Strangely, my biggest worry was that I would go bald. But I reacted differently to the chemotherapy than most people. I did not lose my hair; it just turned all white.

Six months later I got word that I was no longer at risk for more cancer. But I continued to get blood tests and checkups once a month, and not until the fifth year after my initial diagnosis was I finally deemed cancer-free.

During the year of recovering from cancer and being away from my children, I was able to get in touch with my soul. That is when I discovered mandalas, patterns that have a spiritual meaning. In Sanskrit, the word *mandala* means "window to the soul." Its literal meaning is center, circle, and completion.

These days, outlines of mandalas are printed in coloring books for adults because coloring them is calming and healing. When I first started coloring mandalas, engaging in this activity calmed me and allowed me to reflect more deeply. It felt like a gift from the universe, from God. When I started sharing mandalas with other people who were going through hard times, I noticed that this form of engagement also helped them become centered and cultivate a positive mindset that aided healing. So I started to play with mandalas more. I'd ask people, "How about if you attach a question to your mandala and then I'll read the mandala for you?" That idea must have come from the universe. The next thing I knew I was offering spiritual readings using mandalas.

Eventually I found a spiritual leader who showed me how to read colors and be quiet enough to allow information to come through the mandalas. I was amazed at how accurate my readings were. They became a way to soothe my soul and share mandalas with as many people as possible in Hawaii and elsewhere. Having the ability to balance medical, natural, and spiritual aspects is, I believe, my strength and why I am doing what I do today.

Do you feel that your health problems occurred so you would receive the gift of mandalas that you share with other people?

Yes, I believe there was a purpose behind it. Being diagnosed with cancer taught me that I had always been on the go in my life and now needed to take a path of deeper self-awareness and maintain a better balance between mind, body, and spirit. Many people diagnosed with a disease see only the diagnosis. However, it's very important to understand that health is not just a medical issue but has to do with the mind, body, and spirit. When we can bring them together and achieve balance among them, it's amazing the power we have in our lives and what we can accomplish. That's the message I share with others.

It's a beautiful and powerful message. I am curious to understand a little more about how a mandala-making session works with your clients.

As children, we colored for fun. By contrast, mandala coloring for adults is a form of meditation, allowing them to get in touch with their challenges and inner fears. Mandalas are actually a manifestation of who we are. When we color a mandala while emptying ourselves of questions in our minds, the questions are transferred to the mandala, and the results are incredible. Mandalas are used in a lot of spiritual ceremonies all over the world. They bring calmness so people can shift their awareness from their heads to their hearts and align themselves with their spirits to better assess where they are and where they want to go, instead of where they have been. It's amazing how such a subtle shift can take us to a whole different path. Mandalas as tools give us a broader perspective, enabling us to make better decisions and go with the flow.

I've felt the power of mandalas, as well. I colored them when I was going through a rough period. Choosing all the beautiful colors and drawing with the hand led to a profound form of self-expression that was very soothing. How did you know to trust the effects of interacting with mandalas and the messages you got from them?

I believe that my upbringing in Hawaii prepared me for that. It's part of our culture. From an early age, my father and mother would say to me, "Trust your instincts." And we usually can confirm, by doing additional research, that following our instincts brings positive results. I have aunts and uncles who always followed their intuition, and it has never steered them wrong. So such trust was instilled in me from birth. I also learned to trust what comes from interacting with mandalas after seeing how they help people experience oneness, gain clarity about the direction in which they want to go, and make better decisions.

Do you have any advice about how to listen to intuition and how to determine whether you are actually perceiving information coming from your intuition?

The advice I can give to others seeking such knowledge is that when something comes from your head you will always have doubt. But when something comes from your heart and permeates your whole being you can trust that it's from your intuition. With the head, we choose paths based on various reasons. But the heart doesn't reason; it just is. When you can separate from your intellect's constant analyzing and just be, the power you step into is amazing.

Lately I have been seeking advice from financial experts. I have received some smart counsel, but intuitively I got a different message. I found that the minute I started moving in the direction indicated by my intuition everything came together smoothly. Also it seems that at times the end result is not as important as the feedback we get from the experiences we have in each moment.

Absolutely.

Mamie, is there anything else you would like to share?

Just know that when you know, you'll know—and trust that.

WISDOM TO REMEMBER

Mamie-Jean Lamley received the shocking news that she had cervical cancer while teaching people how to think like a leader, presenting qualities she herself exemplified. She did so first by having three children after being told she could not have any, and then by facing cancer courageously while taking important steps to address her diagnosis. For example, she surrounded herself with people who offered loving support. She did research to increase her understanding of her condition and various treatments. She trusted her intuition and maintained belief in a bright future. She combined the wisdom of Western medicine and Eastern medicine to maintain a balance between her body, mind, and spirit. Then through mandalas she learned how to focus on the knowledge coming from her heart rather than her head and, in so doing, found inner peace. Finally, because of her health crisis she learned that she had a gift for reading mandalas, and began using it to help others. These are all steps you can repeat to find success on your path toward health and happiness.

WHAT YOU CAN DO

For a calming and healing experience, select a mandala in a coloring book or create your own, and color it in a comfortable, quiet place, either with relaxing music in the background or while sitting in silence. Have lots of colored pencils or crayons ready. Before drawing, practice the mandala meditation below to help tune in to your intuition and soul.

Mandala Meditation

- Start the music.

- Close your eyes, take a deep breath, and exhale. Repeat three times.

- Visualize the following layers of light surrounding you:

    ~ White light of protection closest to your body

    ~ Violet light around that for connection to the universe

    ~ Indigo or navy blue light around that to enhance contact with your intuition

- Meditate to arrive at the questions you want answered.

- Open your eyes, and on a blank sheet of paper write down two or three questions you would like your mandala to address.

- Draw your mandala from your heart, without thinking about it.

- While concentrating on your finished mandala, reflect on your questions and welcome the answers that arise.

CHAPTER 16

Creating Harmony Within

NATUROPATHIC ENDOCRINOLOGY AND STRESS HEALING

With

CONNIE HERNANDEZ, ND

*"Happiness is when what you think, what you say,
and what you do are in harmony."*

—Mahatma Gandhi

C onnie Hernandez, ND, specializes in functional endocrinology (balancing thyroid, adrenal, and reproductive hormones), adjunctive cancer care, autoimmunity, digestive disorders, and mental/emotional/spiritual counseling at Pacific Naturopathic in Mountain View, California. She graduated from Bastyr University Naturopathic Medical School and has also trained in flower essences and homeopathy. Instrumental in my healing, she was very creative in her approach.

Dr. Connie tell us about somebody you helped after they were told elsewhere that it was not possible to change their condition.

The most irresponsible thing that happens in medicine is telling people that there is no cure for what they have, or that there's no way they can heal. That is never true. Someone who says these things is simply saying they don't know what they can do to help the person heal.

Years ago, a woman came into my office looking like a homeless person, disheveled and not well dressed. I could see that she had difficulty moving, her voice sounded feeble, and she had fatigue, muscle pains, and insomnia. She'd been ill for some time, had a ream of laboratory findings, and had visited most practitioners in the area. She had lists of supplements she'd been prescribed that were appropriate to the conditions she'd been diagnosed with. I could see that she'd been treated well, but nothing had worked for her. After she said, "I've been to everybody, and no one can help me," I was initially doubtful that I could help, mostly because she had given up on the possibility of a cure. I then had an intuitive flash about a flower essence remedy. I gave her a little of the remedy and told her to put three drops under her tongue three times daily and to observe any changes.

She had no faith in this remedy, but when she came back a week later she was completely different—well dressed, well groomed, energetic, and optimistic, with no problems. She believed it was the flower essence that had brought this transformation.

Flower essences are energy medicines and are based on vibration. If there is a vibrational resonance between the flower essence and the person, the essence will help with healing. The trick is to find the perfect flower essence for a given individual. I've found that when I have an intuitive flash about a remedy it is generally a remedy that works well and produces positive results. The art of working with flower essences is to allow intuition to inform reason.

What happened to the woman after her transformation?

I only saw her twice again, mostly for encouragement and affirmation. The remedy awakened her vital force and allowed her to move forward.

We often don't move forward, due to some energetic imbalance. But when we address the subconscious or superconscious mind things can change quickly, an outcome that is far more likely with energy medicines, than with pharmaceutical medicines. We get effects with pharmaceutical medicines, but for instantaneous healing at deep levels, we have to use energy medicine—whether it's homeopathy, flower essences, emotional freedom technique (EFT), or machines that monitor and regulate the flow of energy in the body. Energy medicine is the medicine of the future—Einsteinian physics, not Newtonian physics.

How did you start believing in energy medicine?

I was always fascinated by spiritual healers, by vibrational healing of all kinds, but I didn't have a personal experience with it until I was in medical school. I was pregnant, and had an uncomfortable vaginal infection for which I didn't want to take drugs. A homeopathy professor gave me three homeopathic sugar pellets to dissolve under my tongue. I did not believe this would do anything whatsoever for my condition but saw it as an opportunity to learn something about homeopathy. I took the little pellets; we had some tea; and about fifteen minutes later the doctor asked how I felt.

I realized I was feeling great. She had done an exam previously and seen red and inflamed tissue. The red tissue had now been replaced with pink healthy tissue, and all itching and burning was gone. That was stunning to me. In medical school you are generally in a rational space where you're thinking about cause and effect, pharmacology, and physiology—and homeopathy seems farfetched. But there was no arguing with what had occurred. So I began studying energy medicine, reading books on vibrational medicine, and then becoming involved in spiritual practice, which helped me understand healing on a deeper level.

I understand that you originally explored working in the context of conventional medicine and then transitioned into naturopathy. Would you explain the difference between the conventional Western idea of medicine and the Eastern, or natural healing, methods and how they can support each other?

One of the things we were taught in naturopathic medical school was when to refer patients to conventional medical practitioners, primarily when we see that we cannot help a patient, or when that patient is in danger. It was in the spring semester of my second year of naturopathic school that I learned firsthand that conventional medicine has its place. This was during the birth of my son, who I had conceived with the help of naturopathic medicine. Well into a midwife-assisted home water birth, we learned that my son was lying transverse with the cord around his neck, and that my cervix had closed down. I was transferred to the hospital for a C-section. A very wise conventional doctor told me, "The body in its wisdom closed your cervix down to save both you and your son. Neither of you would have survived a natural birth. Had you had a natural childbirth you and he wouldn't be here today." That was an appropriate hospital transfer for a conventional medical solution.

Very often I find that people are averse to being referred to conventional medicine. I told a patient who had symptoms of appendicitis, "You need go to the ER now," but she replied, "No, I've been there three times before with similar symptoms, and they sent me home each time." I insisted, "I'm sending you to the ER." Within minutes she was on the operating table with a ruptured appendix.

Conventional medicine definitely has its place. And pharmaceuticals often work, though they also often have side effects. The most distinguishing characteristics of naturopathic medicine are that practitioners look for underlying causes rather than just treating symptoms and that they recommend nonharmful remedies, including lifestyle modifications and patient self-care.

How do you find out the cause of someone's condition when they come to your office?

I do a detailed history and review of symptoms, ask questions and listen. You have to think outside the box and listen to your intuition. You may see a complaint on the schedule, but when the patient comes in they often start talking about an emotional issue, and then you know that something else is causing or promoting the symptoms. Of course, we also evaluate both conventional lab tests, though we often interpret them differently from how they are conventionally evaluated, and we make use of alternative methods of testing as well. Because of the way the nation's insurance system works, conventional doctors look for a diagnosis to attach a code to before billing the insurance provider—a diagnosis that may have nothing to do with what needs to be optimized or with what has changed for that person. We always look at sequential comparative lab results. We want to know what's normal for that patient, what changed, and what was happening when the changes occurred.

What questions can people ask themselves to better understand the cause of their health issue?

They could ask themselves, "How do I benefit from this condition?" That's a hard question because it feels to the patient like blaming the victim; but it really involves increasing patient awareness of a potential benefit or what the condition might represent on a subconscious emotional level.

Would you give us an example of that.

For instance, when I went to an orthopedic surgeon for shoulder surgery, the surgeon said he would be shaving away parts of the joint that were impacting each other. It sounded like he would be removing a chip from my shoulder, so I thought, *Do I have an attitude that has created a chip on my shoulder, and will its removal help me attend to changing something about my consciousness?*

This motivated me to look at how I might be harboring resentment and, if so, how I could get rid of such thoughts.

Do you feel different having gotten the chip off your shoulder?

I am not putting the same stress in my shoulder as before, either physically or emotionally. This correlates with not having the same resentful attitudes anymore. You have to look at every angle of a health problem and work with all aspects you discover. That's why we often say that naturopathic medicine is not cookbook medicine.

If I said I've been diagnosed with hypothyroidism, what aspects of it would you look at?

That's a big question because hypothyroidism is routinely misdiagnosed. On a diagnostic level, I would want to know: Is it an autoimmune problem and the thyroid issue is just the result of the autoimmunity? Is it a problem of the brain not telling the thyroid what to do? Is it a problem of the brain telling the thyroid what to do and the thyroid producing thyroid hormone but not converting it to the active form, and if that's true, why? Is it due to injury, adrenal situations, low iron in the system, or nutrient deficiency?

On an energy level, I would note that the thyroid is connected to the throat chakra and communication, so I would want to know if you are able to speak your truth, what kinds of relationships you are having, and what kind of work you do. All those things come into play. I don't say, "You have low thyroid hormone. Let's give you some Synthroid."

Another good example of maintaining a holistic perspective is the view of asthma. If a person's asthma is grief stored in the lungs, I'll give them a homeopathic or a flower essence before giving them anything else. If the asthma is triggered by exercise, I might give them a thousand milligrams of vitamin C three times a day. If it's triggered by allergy, then I'd have to find and treat the allergy. There are many potential reasons for the presence of any particular symptom, and I have to look to those to understand how to treat each patient.

I remember you doing quite a few creative things with me.

You were open to creative things. I have to take into account patient preferences and belief systems. I have patients who only want flower essences; they want to work on a vibrational level with whatever is going on. Other patients might walk out the door if I give them a flower essence or tell them to wear a blue scarf around their neck to stimulate thyroid function.

How would you describe true healing?

Healing comes when patients achieve harmony within themselves. Healing is not necessarily disappearance of the diseased state. A lot of cancer patients have come to us with stage 4 cancers. Many of them will not live but will nevertheless feel like they've experienced healing.

For example, a Pacific Islander with four little kids came to us from Stanford with stage 4 cancer. She'd been treated with chemotherapy, but it hadn't worked, and they'd told her to go home and die. She came in with her huge extended family and begged us to do IV vitamin C for her, which Stanford had refused to do. We turned the clinic upside down to meet all the requirements for doing that in the office. As a result of the treatment, she regained her sense of well-being and was able to spend happy time with her family six months longer. Her family invited us to her memorial service, at which many people expressed their gratitude, saying they felt like she had been healed in the sense that she had had the time to come to peace with herself and her family. The cancer was not healed, but the family was healed. Because of her, we set up an IV center at the clinic and started working with other cancer patients.

I have been taught that disease often comes from stress. What technique would you recommend to help overstressed people in their busy lives?

I recommend breathing exercises as a basis for meditation. I don't know how people with complaints of anxiety, depression, irritability, or insomnia exist in stressful environments without meditation. I don't think such people get better unless they have a way of tuning in to their inner selves.

Would you guide us in the practice you call Ten Conscious Breaths?

It's a very easy practice that only takes two minutes. We're not trying to change the rhythm of our natural breath; we're just trying to observe the breath. Breathe in through the nose and then allow the breath to escape through the mouth. Do this ten times, and you will find that by the tenth breath you are in an altered state of consciousness. If you have elevated blood pressure, you can train for this on a blood pressure cuff: take your blood pressure, loosen the cuff, do ten breaths, then take your blood pressure again. It will likely show drops in systolic and diastolic pressure of ten to twenty points.

You know what? I actually did that once. I had my blood pressure taken and was doing a breathing exercise. The nurse looked worried and asked if I normally have low blood pressure. I replied, "No," but aware of what had just occurred I added, "Why don't you try it again?" This time I chatted with her rather than doing the breathing exercise, and my blood pressure was back to normal.

You can also do this practice to control your digestive enzymes before eating. There are many other reasons to be silent, in a meditative state, or blessing your food before eating a meal. Tuning in to your inner self in these ways vibrationally changes things, relieving tension and bringing you into a state of autonomic nervous system balance.

I often advise people to practice Ten Conscious Breaths in the morning upon waking up, at night before bed, before each meal, and anytime they feel agitated. After doing the practice over a period of time, they may only need one or two breaths to get to a calm state. They will also start to feel where and when they're holding tension, and take care of it to prevent health issues in the future.

WISDOM TO REMEMBER

When doctors say nothing can be done to help people, it just means they have not found a solution. True healing occurs when we achieve harmony within ourselves. At that point, even if a disease does not disappear we can live to the end of our lives with greater happiness, less physical and emotional pain, and the ability to enjoy our loved ones.

Today, we are increasingly seeing the use of energy medicine and tapping into the subconscious and superconscious minds for healing. When deciding on a healing plan, the whole person needs to be considered. Western conventional medicine, Eastern natural healing, and modern healing approaches all have appropriate uses, depending on a person's situation and beliefs. You do not need to fear conventional medicine as it helps save lives. Naturopathic medicine specializes in looking for the underlying causes of health problems, finding nonharmful solutions, and encouraging people to change their lifestyle and practice self-care measures to improve their chances of healing.

WHAT YOU CAN DO

To create a holistic approach to self-healing, ask yourself:

- Did this health issue start on the heels of a challenging emotional situation in my life?

- What meaning or benefit could this health issue have for me?

To reduce stress:

- When feeling anxious, lower your blood pressure by practicing Ten Conscious Breaths, breathing in through your nose and out through your mouth ten times in your natural rhythm, without pushing.

- Each day practice Ten Conscious Breaths upon waking up, before going to bed, and before eating.

To help with digestion:

- Before eating, take a moment of silence to calm your nervous system.

- Practice Ten Conscious Breaths to stimulate your digestive enzymes.

- Bless your food to shift its vibration to match that of your natural state.

CHAPTER 17

Perfect Spirit

ALLEVIATING MULTIPLE SCLEROSIS, BIPOLAR DISORDER, AND SUICIDAL TENDENCIES USING MEDITATION

With

SAM SHELLEY

"Realize deeply that the present moment is all you ever have."

—Eckhart Tolle

Sam Shelley's story is of a man plagued by multiple sclerosis, bipolar disorder, and suicidal tendencies for most of his adult life before he underwent a transformation that made him symptom free in eighteen months. Not only did he heal his body but he discovered how to live joyfully. Author of *I Don't Dwell: How I Used Meditation, Mindfulness and Yoga to Reverse My Incurable Diseases*, he is now a mindset mentor and abundant life strategy consultant.

Sam, would you share your experiences before and after your healing.

My pain and suffering began early in life. At six, I was run over by a van that crushed the whole left side of my body, nearly killing me. I had a slim chance of survival. I almost bled out. I had a lot of trauma and was in the hospital for about a year, then spent four months in rehab.

After the accident, my parents were naturally always worried about me, so I started to obsess about myself. Out of that I became bipolar, though un-diagnosed until my twenties. I had to be institutionalized twice due to being suicidal. I also had to go through a few other things along the way: psoriasis, psoriatic arthritis, and migraines. At age thirty-seven, I lost the ability to walk because of multiple sclerosis (MS), a disease of the brain and spinal cord that affects the nervous system. I had no coordination on the left side of my body, and I was basically blind from optic neuritis for a while. The left eye was jumping around like crazy; the right eye was blurry. I couldn't do much of anything, having lost most of my functions. Today, I take no medicine and use no cane. I'm pretty much a medical miracle.

That's amazing. How did it happen?

One day I was reading a book about meditation that stated "meditation equals inner peace," so I'm like, *I need that.* I began at night with a five-minute practice. The first two weeks were very difficult because I thought the brain was supposed to stop thinking. Instead, I soon realized that the brain never stops thinking, that it's all a matter of how we react to our thoughts and if we believe they are true. After three or four months of meditating—ten minutes in the morning, ten minutes in the evening—one evening I heard a voice say, "Perfect spirit." *That's it,* I realized. *My spirit is perfect, but my body is damaged.* Then I knew that all my health symptoms were simply gone. Encouraged by this inner knowing that all was well, I began to taper off my medicine, which I don't recommend. It took me eighteen months to get off all my medicine. Of course, some of the doctors didn't understand why I was doing this, but I persisted anyway.

My intuitive voice was very loud after that night. I went from having a really chatty mind to having a quiet mind, and my intuitive voice was now guiding my way forward. I just let go of all the stories I had in my head from all these diseases. You read stories about diseases like bipolar disorder and multiple sclerosis; encounter stigmas about being bipolar; and hear people telling you what your diseases should be like. For instance, they say, "You're supposed to be tired all the time. This is supposed to happen, that's supposed to happen." I had all these beliefs that I had to surrender. That's where I focus today because I never had a teacher. I simply trusted my own intuition on letting go and doing what I needed to do.

My intuitive voice also told me that I needed to do yoga, so I did yoga. At first yoga was very tough. I fell over a lot at the beginning, but six months later I didn't need my cane anymore because of all the practice I'd done.

I persistently worked to heal my body because, though my mind wanted another body, I knew I couldn't get one. With meditation things are very peaceful, but it was day-to-day mindfulness that helped me the most—being mindful that the mind is a time traveler. The mind likes to drag us into the past or the future. But all we really know for certain is what's right here in front of us. We have no idea what's going to happen an hour from now. For instance, an hour earlier I thought we were going to be talking on the phone; I wasn't expecting to do a video chat. But that's life, and you just deal with it. Whatever presents itself you deal with it, whereas the mind would say, *Wait, this isn't acceptable.* Right and wrong is all a matter of perspective. I've never done a video call in my car before, so it's like, *All right, where can I mount my phone so it's not jumping all over?* This is going with the flow, not letting the mind cling to anything like, *Oh, I can't do this.*

I had a similar struggle because of the construction that's happening on the outside of my apartment building. I had meetings with the building manager to see about minimizing the noise or putting me somewhere else, but we couldn't find a solution. Then I wondered if we should cancel the interview, but I really wanted to do it now. So I found a spot in my apartment a bit farther from the noise.

You just have to go with the flow of life. You're constantly surrendering with the mind and living for the moment. All we have to be concerned with is this moment.

Yes. Since being off meds, did you get diagnostic feedback from the doctors, affirming that you don't need them?

The last time my neurologist saw me, maybe in 2012, he tried for forty-five minutes to quantify what I did by asking various questions. He remarked that my blood work was better than his and the only thing he saw on my physical exam was a nonspecific hand tremor that most people have. I have had no need for medicine over the five years since then and no ER visits, so something has changed.

Was it when you first heard your intuitive voice say "perfect spirit" that you knew your body would heal, or was that not a thought yet and you just focused more on spirit and then the body healing came as a nice surprise?

I knew at that instant that my health problems were over. Dr. Wayne Dyer calls such times when things become crystal clear "quantum moments." That was my quantum moment, when a quantum shift started me on the mend very quickly.

That's wonderful. It took me four years to get off my medication from the time I started to need a lower dosage. I did work with the doctors in the beginning. Then I worked with an Ayurvedic doctor who intuitively checked my thyroid level so I didn't have to have, and pay for, the invasive blood tests. But after a while I said to that doctor, "I know what's happening with my body and how much to lower my dosage. Could I just do this on my own?" She responded yes. The rest of the voyage I did on my own. It was very special to have that empowerment and to know that we have such potential.

Right, because there's a perfect spirit within everyone. We have everything within us, and our intuitive voices will guide us.

What advice do you have about how to listen to that intuitive voice and be aware of its importance?

That's a tough challenge. How do you distinguish between the mind voice and the intuitive voice? The mind voice is always second-guessing, always critical. It is very assertive and plays the "what if" game: *What if I do this? What if I do that?* The intuitive voice is more supportive and nurturing, and when you hear it you simply know.

It was not an easy ride to get off medicine. I had a lot of withdrawal symptoms, but my intuitive voice reminded me once in a while that no matter what I was facing all was well. The mind always makes you think that whatever is happening in the present is the worst thing, but your intuitive voice can always remind you of a time when things were worse.

How can we use the mind in a positive way?

I see the mind in two ways: it's either dragging you around all over the place or it's full of challenges. I'd say 90 percent of our thoughts are nonsense. The rest are actually supportive and helpful. The nonsense thoughts are theories about yesterday and guesses about tomorrow. We have to use the mind to function in the world, but we don't have to constantly listen to it or pay attention to it.

What actually needs to be healed?

It depends. Sometimes the body gets damaged, and practices such as yoga are needed to restore it. One test that came to me was to look at pictures of myself and realize that the body is temporary. A few days after my quantum moment I was sent some pictures in the mail—baby, toddler, and young teen photos of myself. I looked at these pictures and wondered, *Where did I go?*

I had all these bodies, but my perfect spirit, who sees through the eyes, has never changed. We're constantly getting new bodies. The body is a fragile thing. Stuff happens to it. I'm just fortunate that my body was able to heal itself so much. It's really an odd process. I guess my intuitive voice was telling me that I had to bring my body back to health by doing yoga, taking time for myself, and eating better.

Where did these changes lead you in your life?

Now my life is real interesting because I don't claim to do anything. I call myself an experience junkie. Whatever happens, happens, and I just go with it. If I don't like the way things are going, I change it. Being comfortable with your situation is very easy; jumping into the unknown is a leap of faith. You're constantly making that leap of faith, trusting that all is well. Limitations come in your mind, but once you can let go of them there's nothing you cannot do. Of course, your body may not have the skills to do something without practice; if you want to be a gymnast, obviously you're going to need to practice. But you can do that.

Humans can do all sorts of things with dedication and practice. Nobody just jumps into playing guitar and immediately creates songs and has big hits on the radio. You need time as well as practice. The mind wants instant gratification, but life unfortunately doesn't work that way. You have to put some effort, some kind of intention, into it. Like, I had this intention that meditation equals inner peace, and an inkling I wanted inner peace, so I sat there doing meditation every day. That inner peace came when I heard my intuitive voice. Then a whole bunch of other things came that I wasn't expecting, but I did the act of surrendering.

Do you feel that you could use intention to affect anything in your life? For instance, I can think of the construction workers outside who are using a loud machine, and say, "Operating this loud machine causes inner peace," or I can say, "Jumping out of planes causes inner peace" or "Creating a computer program causes inner peace." Do you feel it's going to have the same effect?

Yeah, you can use intention to create inner peace in any situation. It's important to realize that behind the noise of the world there's always an underlying silence. Similarly, in Taoism the truth that can be spoken is not the great truth; silence is the great truth, and the silence is always there. It's like in a song: if there were no pauses, it would just be a buzz-saw noise, but it's those pauses that give music meaning. That silence is there in music to highlight the notes. Otherwise, they're just part of the noise of the world.

Nice. Would you walk us through a technique that can help us tune in to the intuitive voice and the silence within.

There's all sorts of things you can do. For example, you can close your eyes and touch your legs, realize this is your body, and use the sensation to tune in to the intuitive voice because sensations are always in this moment. When doing this, there's no story—just sensation without judgment. Anytime you judge, you are in the mind. When you just feel the sensation of touching the leg, you are not focusing on problems, just experiencing peace.

That's a great tool for helping bring us into the present moment.

Right. I always find the Dalai Lama interesting to watch. If you notice, he's constantly touching things. Whether it's people or objects, he's engaging his senses. He's not allowing his mind to tell stories. His senses are always in this moment. When you're touching something, the mind has to interpret what you're touching.

That's fascinating. Why do you think we were given a mind?

Well, because it's a tool to deal with the situations and challenges of life. It's either a tool or it can drag us around. Most people let it drag them around. If you look in people's eyes, you can spot those who are not really here. They're listening to the chatter in their minds, trying to understand what's going on instead of just embracing life.

Do we need to process anything?

To go forward in life, sometimes it's helpful to understand a little bit; but most of the time we cannot really understand what's going on in life, or we get stressed trying to figure out why such and such happened. I got really stressed trying to figure out why I was getting all these diseases. So I just let that go since it didn't really matter. The way I saw it when I was bipolar was that there are many bipolars running around doing all sorts of crazy things, but with MS I lost the ability to walk. I saw that the universe gave me a good sign, saying, "You can't run around anymore, so I guess you've got to deal with it and go within." The universe got my attention. I don't see anything as a mistake—it's simply feedback. Are we paying attention to what's going on around us and to our own bodies? Maybe *that's* what we need to process.

Beautiful. Now you've also been able to use your experiences, your knowledge, and your studies to help others. How do you help others pay attention like that?

I just talk to everyone. I see everyone as their own snowflake. All people build their own life experiences. The best example of this occurred when I was in California, where I had a client who really liked watching football, and I made football-watching a spiritual practice to get this man to question his mind. At one point a player was hurt on the field, and I asked my client questions like, "What do you think about that?" and "Why do you think that's true?"

He ended up questioning his own thoughts, asking himself: *How do you know what he's thinking and feeling? How do you know if a thought is really true?* You're constantly questioning your thoughts. Byron Katie does work with questions that have you repeatedly challenging your thoughts and situations—like you think something is true, but is it really true? It's all your perspective.

What transformations have you noticed in the people with whom you've worked?

The biggest transformation I've seen in people I've worked with is that when we begin a session they're usually either neutral or not so happy, and by the time we're done they're happy, laughing. They just need opinions that were bogging them down to go. The work is about bringing people back into the moment so they're not so caught up in the story of life.

That's interesting. When I offer energy healing and tarot readings at expos, I find that people walk away from both with the same expression of relief, healing, and light in their faces. In the tarot readings, all I do is

enable them to shift their perspective or get ideas on how to handle their challenges. Simply shifting the mindset is very healing for people.

It's all about changing perspective, giving people a different way to look at things. There is something else involved, too, that I can't explain. I go into a meditative state, and it's as if Sam goes offline and my intuition speaks through me to people. I get into a silent space and just say words that come through, and the people make dramatic shifts. Eckhart Tolle said that from the silence comes wisdom.

That's really helpful for people to understand because we often feel as if we need to make life be a certain way and make our words follow a certain format. If you were to create a formula that offers security, what formula do you think could work for everyone?

I'd say all the formulas and rules are made up—they're in people's heads. I'd advise people to just find one thing that brings them peace, joy, and happiness and learn to appreciate all the things they can do. I had to lose my ability to walk to get gratitude. When you're helpless, you become thankful for all things. That's why I'm always happy today: I've been through worse times, and now I'm grateful for every little thing. So the one formula is just to be grateful, to appreciate how you are reacting to situations.

There are really only two certain things in life—death and trauma. Everybody's going to die; everybody's going to face trauma, some kind of situation that's going to bring pain. What's important is how you deal with that trauma.

In meditation, we often try to unite with the world around us and expand our awareness. How do you perceive that concept?

For me, meditation was about finding underlying peace. Actually, it was a benefit that I never had a meditation teacher. If I had told my bipolar OCD brain that I had to sit a certain way, hold my hands a certain way, breathe a certain way, I'd have been so focused on the rules that I would have never gotten out of the mind. So not having rules and not having teachers were great benefits for me. I just trusted myself, trusted that I could actually find inner peace.

I come from a path with techniques. Part of the reasoning behind it is that if we didn't have techniques we would continue to experience the pain we normally have and not find a way out. What natural process would you recommend to help people avoid the pains they're feeling?

Many people who start a new meditation practice sit way too long. When you sit too long, the mind gets very busy, very chatty, and the mind voice becomes louder. Meditating one minute a day, on the other hand, makes a huge difference. Then you can add another minute, two minutes, three minutes. A journey of one thousand miles begins with a single step. The mind wants instant gratification, but the only way you can get quiet is gradually—one minute a day and then two minutes a day, and so forth. When the mind gets busy, you need to come back to sensation. Just keep coming back and don't judge. When you constantly return to thoughts, stop for the day and say, "Okay, I'll try again tomorrow. Maybe I can go for a little bit longer tomorrow."

My process, which was mostly silent, was difficult. Silence is the hardest practice because the mind gets very loud and annoying, constantly playing the "what if" game. It's continually rehashing the day or guessing about tomorrow. You just have to find the happy medium that works for you. People come to me who have been doing practices for fifteen, twenty years, and I encourage them to let go of techniques because they've only gotten so far by using them; so I have them let them go completely and walk those last ten feet themselves, without techniques. Probably what's holding them back from total freedom is believing that use of a technique is the only way. But it's not.

At a certain point I also felt that techniques were taking me away from myself versus just being with myself and experiencing the beauty that already existed within. I had to add that time in without techniques or sometimes just drop the techniques. Or if I did the techniques I had to

do them as something fun and feel the sensations in my body while doing them.

Right, that's why I initially began helping people heal, but what I'm really seeing is people coming to me wanting to deepen their spiritual practice. I've had to encourage them to let go of any rituals, any techniques, which they're often not even aware they're following. In helping people with their healing, I also have them take time for themselves, time away from chasing the infinite to-do list in the mind. All those items in the mind aren't going to bring lasting happiness—fleeting happiness, yes, but not lasting happiness.

What brings you lasting happiness?

Knowing that everything is okay, that my spirit will continue regardless of this body.

What's the best way to embrace fear and get over that hurdle into the unknown?

The unknown is scary for a lot of people. They'd rather deal with pain they're comfortable with than jump into the unknown. They have to explore where the fear is coming from. If they're unable to dive into that fear alone, I will dive into it with them and help them explore it and root it out. I had to deal with that myself because of my bipolar diagnosis.

Unfortunately, today bipolar is about medicine or the psych ward. My therapist never suggested meditation. It was always about medicine, but I'm living proof that medicine isn't the answer. If you can surrender enough and trust your own intuition enough, then you can find a way out. You may have somebody help point the way on occasion. What I saw for myself was that meditation wasn't enough, yoga wasn't enough. What was required was daily moment-to-moment mindfulness to keep myself out of the mind.

WISDOM TO REMEMBER

Sam Shelley spent most of his life in pain and disease until he discovered how to relate to the mind through just a few minutes of meditation without any techniques. He proposes that shifting how you use the mind and developing trust in your intuition can completely change the way your body functions. The mind helps you navigate the material world; it does this by reminding you of other people's stories about disease or by catapulting you into the past or future, invariably removing you from your inner experience of the present moment. Trusting your intuition, on the other hand, anchors you in the present moment, which keeps you tuned in to the existence of a perfect spirit within an ailing body and to the abundance of healing wisdom contained within the body itself. We benefit greatly when guided by the intuitive voice in lieu of the mind voice. Remember to focus on what you are grateful for and get to know yourself in silence.

WHAT YOU CAN DO

To tap into your intuitive voice:

- When distracted by the mind voice during meditation or other activities, touching any part of your body will make you instantly aware of sensations, forcing your mind to focus on the body, the present moment, and the intuitive voice.

- When beginning a meditation practice, start with one minute a day then gradually increase to two minutes and longer. This will help prevent your mind from slipping into busyness and slowly train you to get to know yourself.

- If you are an experienced meditator and not feeling benefit from your practice, experiment with dropping all the techniques you have been taught either for the whole practice or at least part of it. Focusing on techniques can keep you caught in the mind. Sitting still and listening can eventually quiet the mind so the intuitive voice can come through.

- If the message you hear starts with "What if," it is the mind voice; if it feels nurturing and supportive, it is the intuitive voice.

CHAPTER 18

Choice

NON-HODGKIN'S LYMPHOMA NEAR DEATH

With

MAUREEN BELLE

"Change will not come if we wait for some other person or some other time. We are the ones we've been waiting for. We are the change that we seek."

—Barack Obama

Maureen Belle is a traditional shaman intuitive, feng shui and gaia-mancy master, author, and green living and architectural building consultant, but none of those titles prepared her for the diagnosis of stage 4 non-Hodgkin's lymphoma. Today she is healthy and vibrant, and happy to share the profound experience that transformed her through her business and book *Conversation with Heaven and Earth: Healing the Pain of Disconnection*.

I find it interesting that you were involved in a number of healing modalities before experiencing non-Hodgkin's lymphoma. I was a yoga and fitness instructor when I was diagnosed with Hashimoto's and hypothyroidism, and most people would think that at the time I was perfectly

healthy so something like that shouldn't have happened. That lead me to understand there's a deeper message behind disease. Maureen, would you share your experience with disease?

For many years, I had a school focused on shamanism and permaculture, where I taught students to connect to the earth. Then in 2006 I was conducting classes all over the world in green design and feng shui. I was also working on my own building project on Whidbey Island. I wasn't feeling well but ignored it.

I got increasingly weaker and ended up in a wheelchair. I was in serious denial because I ate organic food, exercised, focused on health modalities, and was a good person, so I didn't see how I could be ill. Doctors did blood tests and determined things were off, but they weren't sure what was going on. Meanwhile I became anemic and developed shingles. Nothing, including my extensive experience with healing modalities, as well as being a ThetaHealer and Reiki master, prepared me for my diagnosis.

When, in September 2006, I finally collapsed, unable to walk, a friend took me to a hospital. This time the doctors did blood tests and diagnosed me with cancer. I then became immersed in the world of allopathic medicine. I was sent to a hematologist and oncologist, who did exploratory surgery because a CAT scan showed a tumor on my pancreas. Also they did bone marrow tests, which showed cancer cells in my bone marrow, as well as in lymph nodes from my neck to my groin. The doctor in charge pronounced, "I'm sorry, but you're stage four. Get your affairs in order." I was given six to eight weeks to live. My sister took me to her home to die.

I bought into it, which is hard to understand, given all the prior experiences I had had with natural healing modalities. I was admitted to UC Davis for cancer treatment, but they warned me that there wasn't much hope. Months went by as I did chemotherapy and had surgeries to try to remove the tumor, but with no success. They just said, "We're sorry. Prepare yourself to die."

By January, my five-foot-five body weighed eighty-five pounds. I had hospice care and was hooked up to morphine and oxycodone for the pain. I hadn't eaten much in months and was a skeleton, literally wasting away. A Reiki master came to give me massages. And I had acupuncture, during which they would literally pick me up and put me in different places, I was that small.

One day my son visited to say good-bye and to give my sister a break. In the middle of the night while we were talking, he suddenly said, "Mom, I don't get it. You were a single mom who raised me by yourself. You ran your own businesses. What happened? You didn't fight." He left the room, and I thought, *Oh my God, did I have a choice in all this?* Then I realized I had just gone along with the program because the doctors had said I was going to die.

For weeks I had been dreaming about myself walking on a path through the forest, the path I used in my shamanic work. For about two weeks before my son's arrival, there had been two paths and two of me, and I knew this represented my body and soul splitting.

After my son left, I thought, *Okay, I can leave now.* I closed my eyes, and the next thing I knew I was engulfed in light. There was an all-encompassing presence of love: I was the presence, and the presence was me. The pain was gone. I was in complete peace, in balance, in harmony, and I felt a connection with everything in the universe. Then a voice said, "Choice." A presence came forward, and I replied, "Yeah, choice." I realized this presence was saying that if I wanted to I could go back.

I was as shocked as I could be in a blissful state. I looked down, and I was way above my body, which looked like a bump on the bed. Again I said, "Choice," and the presence replied, "You have a choice. You always have choices, in every moment of the day." I immediately saw how disconnected I had been from my body and how that had led to having cancer.

The presence gave me three missions to accomplish if I chose to go back. The first was to teach people to move past the illusion of separation that has harmed humanity and our planet for millennia. The second was to help people understand that their bodies are sentient beings. The third was to realize how important it was that I learn to love humankind as much as I loved nature and animals. I had had a very abusive childhood and had never fully trusted humanity, while I always trusted nature and animals.

Then the presence again said, "Choice." Now I was at about ceiling height looking down at this gray, bald, skeletal body and thinking, *Oh my*

God, go back to that and the pain? Then the presence said, "Well, ask your body." I looked down and realized that my body was still alive in its essence. My soul had separated from it, but it had a life of its own. At that point, I realized our bodies, even in their decomposition, are alive. They're just going back to the earth, where they came from, to join as soul mate with the soul. So I asked my body, "Well, what do you think?" My body replied, "Yeah, let's go for it." So I turned back to the light in utter gratitude and bliss, closed my eyes, and thought, *I'm going to either move further into the light or be back in my body.*

When I again opened my eyes, it was morning, and I was in no pain. I was very weak and emaciated, but I sat up, called into the baby monitor we were using for communication, and my sister came running in. I told her what had happened, and we both started crying, knowing what this meant. Then my stomach started rumbling from hunger. That night I dreamt that I was again one person, body and soul, walking one forest path.

I still had a chemotherapy treatment left, and at first I thought I would not do it, but then I realized I was supposed to do it. During the couple of weeks before treatment, I researched online the derivation of the chemotherapy drugs used in my treatment, plus the myriad of other drugs I'd been given, from prednisone to Neupogen, each with its own side effects. One of the drugs that really struck me was Vincristine, which turns urine red, making me think I was bleeding to death the first time I went to chemotherapy. Significantly, I found out it came from the vinca plant, which I'd been planting all my adult life wherever I lived. I realized the plant was familiar, and that prompted me to establish a personal relationship, a dialogue, with each one of the drugs being used in my treatment. Somehow I knew that doing so was really important. I still chose to have chemotherapy, even though I was starting to eat again, putting on weight, and my hair was growing back. In fact, incredulous about what was happening my oncologist called the infusion centers and asked, "Are you giving her an infusion or a placebo?" They replied, "No, we couldn't give her a placebo."

Usually my body was very resistant to such toxins, and it had usually taken nine or ten hours for me to go through the five drugs they gave me.

Now it took only three. I realized that I had turned poison to nectar by communicating with the drugs being used in my treatment.

After discovering that we have the ability to transmute toxins, I started dialoguing with the remnants of cancer to learn from them. I learned that it was a virus, and I was able to say, "leave" and know what I needed to do to heal. I also learned that the guiding force behind it all was my body—my sentient body that had a life force, intelligence, and life plan of its own, and which joined with me at conception to have this human experience. I realized, too, that my body was my soul mate. We're always searching for our soul mates outside ourselves, never understanding that they are already with us. We'll always be longing until we reconcile with our true soul mates, our bodies.

After these realizations, I started regaining my appetite and putting on a little more weight, but eating was still very difficult to do. Because I had not eaten in months, I couldn't even chew and had no saliva. I considered what I could do. My body said, "Hey, cooking shows." So my sister and I started watching the cooking network TV. As soon as I began salivating she would rush and cook whatever stirred my juices. That's how my body and I found a fun way to get my appetite going.

I was in a wheelchair for a year and then used a walker for another year, all the while dialoguing with my body in the new way I had discovered. The doctors had told me I was going to have a heart defect, the brittle bones of a ninety-year-old, and eventually some other cancer. But now, ten years later, I am very healthy, with strong bones and a robust heart. In fact, I learned how to heal my heart, and I now teach people how to connect with both the physical heart and the heart chakra to heal them. I learned something else, just as important, about the body. Although I had hated my body for letting me down by getting cancer, I realized this attitude was not right and contributes to disease.

The curious thing about disease is that it can get even worse because of our response to it.

Absolutely. I used to call humanity a cancer on the planet. Well, hello, self-fulfilling prophecy. As a result of having a disease, I started teaching interspecies communication in a new way. I had previously taught people how to dialogue with their animals and plants and nature, but after healing I also taught them how to dialogue with their bodies.

I started taking people on a journey to love and honor their bodies. I walked away from my previous career in architectural green design to create a healing, Shamanic and coaching practice to help others heal the pain of disconnection. My intention was to help people dialogue with their bodies as soul mates. When we do that, the longing for anything outside ourselves stops because we feel complete.

Does a person have to have a near-death experience to discover and embrace the sorts of realizations you experienced?

Absolutely not. I found that the people I'm working with usually experience a call from the soul or body and it's generally not prompted by a near-death experience. I tend to have extreme lessons, which I now have decided I don't need to do anymore to learn. It's as simple as just dialoguing with the voices of our bodies.

I've worked as a mediator and guide with people with cancer, fibromyalgia, and multiple sclerosis, to help them dialogue with their bodies in order to reconcile with and honor them. As a result, over the last ten years I have come to love humanity as much as I love nature and animals. Learning who people are through their hearts and communicating with them through their hearts has allowed me to see the good in the majority of humanity. Ninety-nine percent of humanity is good—a beautiful thing.

An idea I've been exploring lately is that the disease occurring in our physical bodies is a message not just about our own bodies but about what is happening with people close to us and often about the planet. Would you share a little more about how you feel the body is connected to the world and to the people around us?

Absolutely. I've written books on feng shui and gaiamancy. There is a universal language that we all can tap in to and use to talk to anything—the chair in an office or the planets in our solar system. We all have that ability.

When we dissolve the illusion of separation that's been fostered for thousands of years, the world shifts from black and white to Technicolor. The world becomes full of unlimited possibilities and incredibly beautiful, compassionate, and loving. We start seeing those qualities in everything around us. That was a big part of my personal transformation, but I couldn't perceive the world this way until I connected with and honored my body. I was having great dialogues with people's pets; but I wasn't talking to my own body, so I wasn't having a full experience.

We do not have to have a traumatic experience for this to happen. It's as simple as dialoguing with and affirming our bodies. They have waited their whole lives to reconcile with us in this manner.

Sometimes people want a formula for how to maintain the health of their bodies and how to heal when they have disease. Is there a blueprint for healing and health?

I guess there is a blueprint, but it's different for each person, just as it is for each building. And just like each person has a specific blueprint of who they are, so does their body. But we're all connected to the same source, which is the blueprint for healing. The body knows what it needs and how to heal itself. But generally we override our receptivity to its messages through our attitudes, thoughts, and practices.

I want to add that our bodies are not immortal—though they do return to the substance of the earth and stardust they came from—but they have their own life plan, intelligence, and destiny. What terminally ill people with whom I've worked have discovered is that their bodies are done and ready to go. Once they're on board with that, they transition peacefully and gracefully without struggle. It's not about longevity or immortality; it's about living the life we came to live fully, with enjoyment and prosperity.

I help people discover these truths. I am just their guide: I help them find the way to proceed and then I step back because they must establish their own relationships with their bodies and their diseases.

I'm finding more often than not that these diseases are viruses, and that it is possible to dialogue with them. Our bodies have complete knowledge of how to fight every virus we may have. In my own healing I've used a lot of herbs and done a lot of juicing. I had no muscle, so I had to find healthy ways to bring my body back using my body as a guide. It told me exactly what to eat, when to eat, and how to eat. It didn't urge me to follow any specific rules, such as to be vegan.

I have heard people describe autoimmune disorders as the body "attacking" itself, or cancer as the body being "confused." What do you think about these descriptions?

Our bodies are never confused. It's our minds that are confused, our mental minds. If we instead think through our heart minds, then we will think very differently. I picture the mental mind like a mouse detached from the computer but not the mainframe, which is the heart mind. If people ask questions of their heart minds, they get very different answers from those they get from their mental minds.

The mental mind is the origin of allopathic medicine. There are amazing doctors, nurses, and practitioners in the allopathic medical system. It's the system itself that's flawed, not necessarily people. For one thing, it is monetary based—something I learned quickly while undergoing my more than million-dollar treatment.

Yes. There's nothing necessarily wrong with money. But we need to look at the big picture when seeking measures that will be supportive of everyone and this planet over time.

In 1999, whales and dolphins, who have been my guides for many years, especially North Pacific humpbacks, showed me that there will be a tsunami of love traveling the planet, driven by the human heart. They explained, "It's going to start in the Middle East." When the Arab Spring happened, I saw the beginning of this movement of energy from human heart to human heart across the planet. As we look past mainstream media, which is based on fear, and see the everyday acts of kindness that happen—including the thousands that occur around us every moment of the day—we realize that the media is causing the illusion of discord. I have great hope for humanity now.

I never would have said that in the past, when I called humanity a cancer on the planet. The immensity of the human heart, the ability we have to heal and love, and our capacity for compassion go beyond anything we've ever been taught. In embracing that, and holding it in our hearts, we heal ourselves and the people around us.

WISDOM TO REMEMBER

Maureen Belle's experience with non-Hodgkin's lymphoma, due to the wisdom she gained as a result of it, ended up being a gift. Despite all her previous knowledge about healing, her dreams and a near-death experience gave her additional insights into how to heal the body. Early in her illness she saw a separation between soul and body, but then she came to view the two as soul mates. She realized she needed to communicate more with her body and love it as a sentient being since it had the wisdom to heal her.

Maureen reminds us that healing is an intuitive progression that follows the blueprint of our individual bodies and souls. Our responses to food and medical treatments change depending on our relationships with them and with our bodies. And while our bodies have individual blueprints we still have a connection with the universe. Your greatest task in healing is to listen to the wisdom of the body and follow its cues. Your next greatest task is to learn to be at peace with what both the body and soul want so healing can occur more quickly and gracefully. That healing may mean the body returns to its full functioning as a human or returns to the earth and separates from the soul.

You need not have a near-death experience to establish clear communication with your body; you can establish a dialogue with it based purely on honor and love for it.

WHAT YOU CAN DO

To help communicate with your body as your soul mate:

- Calm your mind by taking three deep breaths.

- As you breathe in and out, direct your breath to your heart, connecting to it more deeply with each breath.

- Keeping your attention focused on your heart, ask your body's voice to come forward. You will have a feeling, or body sensation. Be present and know you have made a deep connection with your body.

Conclusion

The wide variety of perspectives on healing and healing methods shared in this book reflects the fact that there are many resolutions to people's health challenges. Whether you utilize allopathic medicine, naturopathy, nutrition, physical therapy, sound, light, air, energy, drawing, or meditation, making changes in lifestyle and outlook can help you achieve a more balanced and stress-free life. Even making just one change that we believe in and enjoy can result in better health and increased happiness. It is crucial to remember that fatal pronouncements do not have to be your fate.

Healing happens for those who are:

- Constantly in pain

- Continually fatigued

- Losing their hair

- Repeatedly having migraines

- Overweight

- Constipated or having diarrhea

- Nauseous and throwing up

- Unable to move their arms and legs

- Diagnosed with cancer, diabetes, stroke, chronic pain, chronic fatigue, ADHD, obesity, allergies, blindness, Lyme disease, Hashimoto's, hypothyroidism, multiple sclerosis, bipolar disorder, lupus, cerebral palsy, fibromyalgia, anxiety, parasites, hepatitis C, bird flu, and non-Hodgkin's lymphoma

- Taking medications

- Told their condition is terminal

Healing happens when you:

- Focus on your reason to live

- Listen to your doctor

- Don't listen to everything, like fatal pronouncements

- Get a different doctor

- Conduct your own research

- Stop labeling the disease

- Search for the source behind your symptoms

- Change your diet

- Start to meditate

- Do what you can do

- Let family and friends support you

- Ask what is the gift?

- Learn to be positive

- Believe more is possible

- Look past the physical body

- Bypass the mind

- Heal your emotions

- Align with your divine design

- Listen to your body

- Follow your intuition

- Come from the heart

- Focus on the light

- Have hope

- Realize you have a choice

- See how perfect you are

- Stay in the present moment

- Love yourself

- Do what you love

- Share your "sweet song" or story

Ultimately, true healing is a state of mind beyond the immediate concerns of physical health, something I witnessed at the time of my mother's death. She had been diagnosed with terminal cancer around the same time I was diagnosed with Hashimoto's and hypothyroidism. People say it takes seven years for all the cells in the body to rejuvenate. In seven years my body healed, right before my mother passed away. In her final days, I saw a woman who had been afflicted with many emotional and physical pains in her life suddenly become a joyful child with no concerns. It was then I realized that true healing is learning to be happy no matter what is happening in our lives.

Notes

FOREWORD

1. https://www.cancer.gov/about-cancer/understanding/statistics.

MESSAGE FROM THE AUTHOR

1. http://health.usnews.com/health-news/patient-advice/articles/2016-09-27/the-danger-in-taking-prescribed-medications.

2. http://articles.mercola.com/sites/articles/archive/2011/10/26/prescription-drugs-number-one-cause-preventable-death-in-us.aspx.

3. http://www.npr.org/sections/health-shots/2013/09/20/224507654/how-many-die-from-medical-mistakes-in-u-s-hospitals.

CHAPTER 1

1. https://www.verywell.com/why-are-so-many-people-getting-thyroid-disease-3233167.

2. http://www.motherjones.com/environment/2015/11/dairy-industry--milk-federal-dietary-guidelines/.

3. https://saveourbones.com/osteoporosis-milk-myth; http://www.slate.com/articles/briefing/articles/1999/08/got_osteoporosis.html.

4. Robert Young, *The pH Miracle* (New York: Grand Central Life and Style, 2010), 95, 96.

5. http://www.cnn.com/2016/07/01/health/everyday-chemicals-we-need-to-reduce-exposure-to/index.html.

6. http://lowthyroiddiet.com/low-thyroid-chemicals.htm.

7. http://www.molecularhydrogenfoundation.org/.

8. http://www.be-n-balance.com/tag/benefits-of-alkalinity/.

9. Young, *The pH Miracle,* 120.

10. https://goop.com/wellness/health/the-mysteries-of-the-thyroid/

11. http://health.usnews.com/health-news/patient-advice/articles/
     2016-09-27/the-danger-in-taking-prescribed-medications;
     http://www.npr.org/sections/health-shots/2013/09/20/224507654/
     how-many-die-from-medical-mistakes-in-u-s-hospitals.

12. http://liveanddare.com/benefits-of-meditation/;
     https://www.ncbi.nlm.nih.gov/pmc/articles/PMC2211377/.

About the Author

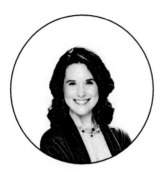

Avital Miller is known for inspiring people to experience boundless energy, absolute happiness, and true success in order to live the best life possible. For over fifteen years Avital has been serving thousands of people worldwide as an award-winning international keynote speaker, healing breakthrough facilitator, and global dancer. Her leadership background includes working as a program manager at Microsoft, lead coach for Success Resources America, sales and marketing director for Crystal Clarity Publishers, yoga and fitness teacher trainer, and fitness director. Her articles have been published in *Fitness Professional Online*, *30 Seconds*, and *Sacred Dance Guild Journal*. She has performed and taught dance internationally since 1993. A graduate of Washington University in St. Louis, Missouri, with a bachelor of science degree in mechanical engineering and a major in dance, she is known for offering beyond-cutting-edge wisdom with authenticity, delightful energy, and infectious joy.

To connect with Avital, hire her for speaking engagements, and participate in her online and live events, please visit www.avitalmiller.com.

Healing Happens

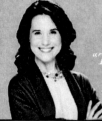

"There are more healing possibilities than we have known."

—Avital Miller

Visit **healinghappensforyou.com** to discover the latest wisdom and techniques for a healthy, happy, and successful life from some of the world's best healing practitioners. Learn simple do-it-yourself natural healing systems utilizing the physical, energetic, mental, emotional, and spiritual layers of healing. Access additional resources and connect with the healing practitioners from the book *Healing Happens*.

Here are some of the healing resources Avital Miller provides for you at healinghappensforyou.com:

- *Online Courses and Webinars*
- *Weekly Podcast*
- *Insightful Blog*
- *Guided Meditations*
- *Energizing Media Clips*
- *Healing Experts' Favorite Books*
- *A Community to Share Your Story*

Plus:

- *Other Healing Resources*
- *Free Gifts, Discounts and Newsletter*

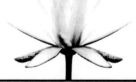

Testimonials from those who have participated in Avital Miller's healing programs:

"I feel more whole and capable of living genuinely in all parts of my life."

—Janet

"This really helped me to look within, value myself, and help me focus on me, and from there be able to take care of others."

—R.M., Vacaville, CA

Gain power over your health and healing, and live a fulfilling life!
www.healinghappensforyou.com

CPSIA information can be obtained
at www.ICGtesting.com
Printed in the USA
FFOW02n0542200618
47152226-49740FF